CLINICAL EXAMINATION ROUTINES, COMMON SIGNS AND SYMPTOMS.

Lecture Notes

A Handy Reference for Medical Herbalists and Complementary Medicine Health Practitioners

Peter Farrell BSc. MNIMH

Copyright © 2017 P. FARRELL
ISBN-13: 978-1543152432
ISBN-10: 1543152430

Dedicated to my kind Mum and Dad, Nellie and Jack, and all parents. May they have happiness and be free from suffering.

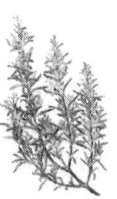

Special thanks to Nancy, my resolutely positive and supportive partner in life.

Thanks to my dear friend and excellent Homoeopath, Kevin Morris, whose words of encouragement, treatments, and example of personal responsibility for one's own health has sustained me in moments of doubt.

Deep gratitude to Marjorie Curtis, who, all those years ago, at the University of Central Lancashire, gave me a chance!

TABLE OF CONTENTS

PREFACE   1

CLINICAL SKILLS DEFINED   3

1. CLINICAL EXAMINATION: GENERAL APPROACH   4

2. EXAMINATION OF THE ORAL CAVITY   7

3. EAR EXAMINATION   10

4. LYMPH NODE EXAMINATION   13

5. CARDIOVASCULAR EXAMINATION   18

    5.1 ESTIMATION OF JVP   27

    5.2 OPTHALMOSCOPY (FUNDOSCOPY) – CVS   30

6. RESPIRATORY EXAMINATION   33

7. ABDOMINAL EXAMINATION   41

8. MUSCULOSKELETAL EXAMINATION   50

    8.1 CERVICAL SPINE   50

    8.2 THORACIC AND LUMBOSACRAL SPINE   53

    8.3 KNEE EXAMINATION   56

    8.4 SHOULDER EXAMINATION   59

    8.5 HIP JOINT EXAMINATION   62

    8.6 ELBOW EXAMINATION   64

9. NEUROLOGICAL EXAMINATION   66

    9.1 MOTOR ASSESSMENT   67

    9.2 SENSORY ASSESSMENT   76

    9.3 COORDINATION   81

    9.4 DEEP TENDON REFLEX   83

    9.5 CRANIAL NERVE EXAMINATION   84

10. KIDNEY AND URINARY TRACT   89

APPENDIX 1. IDENTIFICATION OF PULSES   96

APPENDIX 2. BLOOD PRESSURE   101

BIBLIOGRAPHY   109

Years ago, my mother used to say to me, "In this world, Elwood, you must be oh so smart or oh so pleasant." Well, for years I was smart. I recommend pleasant.

Elwood P. Dowd.

PREFACE

The following set of lecture style notes have been developed from a clinical examination module I delivered as part of the BSc. Herbal Medicine degree course at the University of Central Lancashire. They are meant as a quick reference and general guide for the student herbalist and serve as a simple reference to aid diagnosis but also as an aide-memoir for more experienced herbalists who may not always get the opportunity to practice, and thus recall, rarely used examination techniques. The note style format might also serve as a useful template or support literature for an appropriate clinical examination skills module.

To this end, I have divided the text into distinct areas of examination related to organs and organ systems, although there is some overlap between systems. Each topic has a brief introduction, followed mostly by bulleted points that outline a system of clinical examination techniques along with summarised signs and symptoms that might indicate certain pathologies. The assumption is that the reader will have a sound knowledge of anatomy and physiology, be familiar with some pathology and have a basic idea or introduction to clinical examination.

For fear of overcomplicating an accessible, note style approach and turning it into a textbook, I have avoided the use of instructional photographs and diagrams, except for simplified diagrams, for example, to understand the origin of JVP and to provide easy visualisation of heart sounds, pulse and blood pressure. The routines and diagnostic indications suggested are by no means definitive and do not reflect the extent of clinical examination techniques and diagnosis required in orthodox medicine, but it is hoped that they will function as a quick, general reference/aide-memoir for Herbalists and a support to their 'traditional' system of diagnosis; thus, engendering safe differential assessment.

Although the text is a synthesis of just some of the wealth of knowledge kindly imparted to me by my teachers, many fine herbalists (and beautiful people), not least of all Dr Midge Whitelegg, Graeme Tobyn and Alison Denham, they are heavily based on clinical knowledge and techniques taught to me by Jo Nasr and Janet Wilby; down to earth, no-nonsense practitioners whose character and skills I continually try to emulate.

So here is my offering for what it is worth. Any errors are my own and not that of my teachers. Should the reader note any errors please let me know and I shall endeavour to correct them in future publications.

I hope that you find the contents of this brief guide useful. If you wish to extend your knowledge in this area, I can recommend two detailed and accessible texts on orthodox clinical examination and diagnosis: Bates Guide to Clinical Examination and Clinical Skills by Cox and Roper.

CLINICAL SKILLS DEFINED

In general, we might say that Clinical Skills are comprised of:

1. Case history - Evaluating the patient's symptoms.

2. Clinical examination – Identifying signs and symptoms.

3. Investigation - Biochemical signs, etc.

4. Treatment based on findings of 1, 2 and 3 (diagnosis).

Proficiency in clinical skills results from hard work and experience gained over time. The following lecture notes will provide information mostly on Clinical Examination. Clinical Examination provides information about:

1. The diagnosis of causes of the patient's condition (mostly supporting or eliminating aspects of diagnosis based on case history).

2. The severity of the condition

The following guide is specifically concerned with Clinical Examination – Identifying signs and symptoms.

1. <u>CLINICAL EXAMINATION: GENERAL APPROACH</u>

As most patients on their visit to you will be concerned about their condition and unsure of who you are or of your ability to help them, it is important to immediately generate warmth, genuine concern and confidence. The following provides a general approach to orthodox clinical examination but the same template can be applied to your own chosen tradition with appropriate adaptation.

Conventional method

- Introduce yourself to your patient in an appropriate manner with a warm smile. You might say something like, "Hello Mr Smith I am Peter, the student herbalist, shall I call you Mr Smith...?" (But only if you are called Peter and only if the patient is called Mr Smith!). The diligent practitioner will be aware of 'obvious' signs and symptoms in this first stage of the consultation. The introduction is then, most importantly, followed by taking the patient's case history. At the end of this, if necessary, the clinical examination takes place.

- At an appropriate juncture, prior to physical examination, wash your hands.

- Explain to the patient that you wish to carry out a specific examination. This may be in the form of a request, e.g. If you are carrying out a respiratory examination ask "Do you mind if I examine your hands and have a listen to your chest" and, if not already clear to the patient, explain why you wish to do so. Do not confuse the patient by saying, "I would like to examine your chest" and then immediately proceed to look at the hands. Avoid using medical terms, e.g. "I would like to examine your respiratory system".

- Should the patient agree to your request, give clear directions about how you wish them to be positioned for the examination, e.g. "I would like to examine you on the couch". If appropriate, assist them.

- Carry out any given techniques that will make the patient confident and comfortable and make your examination more effective, e.g. Lying supine for abdominal examination may be uncomfortable for a patient with a low back problem. Placing a pillow under the head and knees will make the patient more comfortable and in addition, will allow examination of a more relaxed abdomen.

- Conventionally, examinations should be carried out in the following general order but this can and should be adapted to each set of clinical circumstances:

INSPECTION-PALPATION–PERCUSSION-AUSCULTATION

- Conventionally, wherever possible and appropriate, work from the patient's right side (This ensures you are always facing the patient, but of course, if you are left handed, it might be best to position yourself on the left).

- First, observe the patient's general demeanour, and inspect the hands and face etc. (Be considerate and gentle, but look and feel like you know what you are doing).

- Having asked the patient to expose only the necessary areas for examination (always being concerned about their modesty), begin palpation followed by percussion and auscultation.

- Before you percuss and palpate, explain to the patient what you wish to do, again ask their permission and encourage them to let you know if something is uncomfortable, tender or painful. Of course, as you examine the patient you will be observing their facial expression and feeling for guarding (a protective, reflex muscular contraction surrounding an area of injury).

- When palpating, do not dig and poke but use careful, firm pressure with rhythmic movements.

- Try to visualise each organ in the region you are examining.

- Keep the patient informed of what you are doing throughout the examination, making further requests when necessary.

- Upon completion of the examination, wash your hands.

General points

- The methods learned as a student are generally suitable for a complete examination and in addition, provide a sound, systematic basis for learning. However, in the clinical setting the method and techniques you use will be dependent on the case history and the particular circumstances.

- The techniques you will learn are tried and tested; to become proficient, you must practice them as they are taught. Undoubtedly, you will be taught alternative techniques by different clinicians, you should take these on board and utilise them if they are more suitable. However, ensure you know why you are using alternative techniques and can explain any reasons for this preference. Variations in technique are not necessarily contradictory or incorrect, they might simply reflect an individual clinician's training and background, or perhaps, be a superior technique.

- It is important to practice the techniques you learn <u>as much as possible</u> on <u>healthy</u> individuals because when you are familiar with normal findings you will be more able to recognise when something is abnormal.

- Know the structure and function of the organs you are examining and the positions they occupy in the body.

The following notes are provided as an aid to learning. Although some instruction is included in the text, there is no substitute for verbal and practical instructions by a qualified herbalist or other clinician.

2. **EXAMINATION OF THE ORAL CAVITY**

Examination of the oral cavity mainly consists of inspection, you might require a tongue depressor and torch/pen-torch. Patients are often a little embarrassed when asked to "open wide", sometimes it helps if you demonstrate it first, e.g. "like this". A good inspection can often take time so, if necessary, allow the patient to rest.

INSPECTION – WHERE TO LOOK AND WHAT TO LOOK FOR
(See Bates: Table 7.18 – 7.21 for abnormalities)

- **Lips** – Colour, moisture, lumps, ulcers, cracking.

- **Oral mucosa** – Colour, ulcers, white patches.

- **Gums and teeth** – Colour, swelling, ulceration.

- **Tongue and floor of mouth** – Ask the patient to put out their tongue - inspect for symmetry (deviation may indicate a CN XII issue, looked at later). Inspect for colour, swelling, white patches, ulcers or nodules - if long term, suspect malignancy; cancers occur most often at the side of the tongue and base of mouth.

- **Pharynx** – Ask the patient to open their mouth and say "ah". If you cannot see the pharynx use a tongue depressor (take care not to cause gagging). Note the rise of the palate (deviation may indicate a CN X issue, looked at later). Inspect the pharynx for redness, enlarged tonsils, and white exudates etc.

Tip
A useful technique to use with patients who tend to be unable to expose the pharynx is to ask them to look at the back of their own throat in a mirror. The pharynx then usually opens suitably for inspection.

SOME FINDINGS ON THE LIPS

- Blue discolouration – Peripheral cyanosis (may be just poor circulation/cold). If noted, always check the tongue for central cyanosis - a grave sign/emergency.

- Dry lips – Weather damage? Dehydration (along with other signs such as dry mouth, loss of skin turgor, dizziness)?

- Swellings - Start of cold sore (followed by blisters and scabs)? Trauma? Cancer?

- Cracking at the sides of mouth (*angular stomatitis*) – Anaemia? Avitaminosis? Excess salivation due to ill-fitting dentures? *Candida* overgrowth?

SOME FINDINGS ON THE TONGUE

- Smooth tongue i.e. absence of papillae (might be swollen, bright red, or fissured) – Iron deficiency? Avitaminosis (riboflavin B_2, niacin B_3, folate, pyridoxine B_6)? Anaemia?

- Thick white coat with underlying erythema – *Candida albicans*?

- Strawberry tongue - White coating covers the dorsum of the tongue with projecting reddened papillae giving an appearance of a strawberry; found in the early stages of scarlet fever (Streptococcal infection, aka. Scarlatina).

- Raspberry tongue - A red, uncoated tongue, with elevated papillae, as seen a few days after the onset of the rash in scarlet fever.

SOME FINDINGS ON THE ORAL MUCOSA

- Redness and vascularity of pillars, uvula and pharynx – Suggests pharyngitis caused by virus (e.g. Epstein-Barr) or bacteria (e.g. *Streptococcus*). NB. Absence of fever, exudate or cervical lymphadenopathy limits the diagnosis of glandular fever.

- Thick white coat with underlying erythema – suggests *Candida*.

- Koplik's spots (small red spots with white centre on buccal mucosa - opposite first and second molars) – Suggests Rubeola, especially if accompanied by fever, coryza and cough.

- Ulcers – Painful apthous ulcer (common) – (increased risk of Ulcerative Colitis in some cases of recurrent apthous ulcer)? Severe neutropaenia (decrease of neutrophils reduces immunity to infection)? Painless ulcer - possible squamous carcinoma? Long standing ulcer or lump - cancer?

SOME FINDINGS ON THE TONSILS

- White exudates – Suggests streptococcal tonsillitis (accompanied by beefy-red uvula and palatal petechiae).

- Thick grey adherent exudate – Consider diphtheria tonsillitis.

- Greyish discolouration of tonsillar tissue – Suggests infective mononucleosis (glandular fever, aka Epstein-Barr virus).

- Red tonsil, protruding forward and medially – Quinsy (peri-tonsillar abscess) which is accompanied by pain, difficulty opening the mouth (trismus) and swallowing, and foetid breath.

3. <u>EAR EXAMINATION</u>

To examine the ear canal (external auditory meatus) and drum (tympanic membrane) requires the use of an **otoscope** using the largest **speculum** the canal will accommodate.

- Position the patient so they are **secure** and **comfortable** and where you can hold and see through the otoscope **comfortably** and **safely**.

- Explain to the patient what you are going to do and that it is normally painless (*when examining infants, you may need to demonstrate on Mum or Dad first*). Instruct the patient to keep their head still during the examination (*when examining infants, it might be helpful to ask Mum or Dad to cuddle them and caress the infant's head to their chest – but NOT put them in a headlock!*).

- For a clear view of the drum, straighten the ear canal by gently pulling the auricle upward, backward and slightly away from the head. (*When examining children, pull auricle downward and backward*).

- Ideally, hold the otoscope between your thumb and fingers (right hand for right ear, left hand for left ear), secure the ulnar side of your hand against the patient's head as you insert the speculum slightly down and forward. Do not insert too deep and avoid pressure on bony areas as this may cause pain.

- If the case history causes you to suspect infection, inspect the non-infected side first to avoid transmission of infection.

<u>SOME FINDINGS IN THE AUDITORY CANAL</u>
(See Bates: Table 7.16 for some abnormalities)

- **Exostosis** – Non-malignant, non-tender nodular swellings on the canal.

- **Chronic otitis externa** – Thickened, red, itchy skin.

- **Acute otitis externa** – Swollen, narrowed, moist, pale and tender and often red.

- **Foreign bodies** – Be careful not to impact it when inserting the speculum.

- **Cerumen** – Ear wax.

SOME FINDINGS ON INSPECTION OF THE EARDRUM
(See Bates: Table 7.16)

- **Normal**
  - Translucent, shiny and pearly grey membrane. It should be free from tears or breaks.

- **Abnormal**
  - Pink, red or bulging membrane indicates inflammation. May find a dull or absent light reflex – Otitis media?

  - Retracted eardrum (showing prominent short process and handle of malleus) - Barotrauma? Eustachitis?

  - White colour indicates pus behind the eardrum.

  - Dull or bluish colour might indicate blood behind the eardrum.

  - Amber fluid behind the eardrum indicates serous effusion - Otitis media? Barotrauma?

PERI-AURICULAR TENDERNESS

- Movement of the auricle may be tender in otitis externa but not in otitis media.

- Tenderness behind the ear may be present in otitis media.

- Exquisite tenderness over the mastoid area suggests mastoiditis. Might be accompanied by a forward protrusion of the auricle.

Note

When the patient complains of pain in the ear (*otalgia*) and examination of the canal and eardrum is normal, suspect referred pain, e.g. Temporomandibular joint (TMJ) dysfunction? Impacted third molar? Periodontal abscess?

4. **LYMPH NODE EXAMINATION**

The Lymphatic system helps maintain the dynamics of tissue fluid exchange and as such aids the removal of excess fluid within tissues. Any pathology which prevents or inhibits the forward movement of lymph fluid in lymphatic vessels will result in a build-up of tissue fluid known as **oedema**.

As part of this process of fluid exchange, lymph fluid aids in the clearing of tissues of waste, toxins and infectious organisms. The nodes within the system of vessels drain locally associated areas of tissue and test for the presence of foreign particulate matter in that fluid, which, if detected, produces an immune response within them, which can result in enlargement or **lymphadenopathy**. Knowledge of nodes and the areas of drainage can aid diagnosis.

EXAMINATION TECHNIQUES

- Ensure the patient's muscles and tendons are as relaxed as possible to facilitate palpation.

- In general, use the pads of the fingers; only use the tips to get a better feel.

- Use the middle three fingers to palpate the clavicular fossa and the tip of the index finger between the heads of the mastoid.

- Examine the cervical nodes separately on each side to avoid bilateral palpation of the carotid sinus, which may cause fainting.

- Submandibular nodes require the use of the middle three fingertips.

GENERAL

- Enlarged nodes anywhere may be due to either generalised or local disease.

- Lung disease tends to spread via the lymphatics to the supraclavicular nodes especially between the heads of the sternomastoid.

- Cancer affecting the stomach and pancreas may particularly affect the left supraclavicular nodes (Virchow's nodes).

- Enlarged nodes higher up the neck is most commonly due to local infections (particularly throat).

- **Normal findings**
  o Normal nodes are not palpable (although small, mobile, soft, non-tender nodes are not uncommon).

- **Abnormal findings**
  o Enlarged mass – tender, warm nodes indicate inflammation or infection.

  o Non-tender, hard nodes might indicate malignancy.

  o Non-tender, soft, matted nodes, cool to touch might indicate TB.

INSPECTION OF THE HEAD AND NECK

With the patient's chin raised and head tilted slightly back, compare both sides and look for apparent enlargement. In general, one can say that nodes are normal or abnormal.

- **Normal**
  o Not visible.

- **Abnormal**
  o Enlarged mass – Infection? Malignancy? Benign mass?

PALPATION OF THE HEAD AND NECK

When palpating, the patient should be relaxed, with the neck flexed slightly forward (if necessary toward the side of the examination). Use the pads of the index and middle finger, or middle three fingers and gently palpate in a circular motion for lymphadenopathy of the head and neck.

SOME INDICATIONS OF ENLARGED NODES IN THE HEAD AND NECK
(See Bates p.203 for position of nodes in head and neck)

- *Supraclavicular nodes* – Important when suspecting intra-abdominal or intra-thoracic structure pathology - tumours may metastasise to these nodes.

- *Cervical nodes* – Viral URT infections? - usually non-tender; Glandular fever? - may be quite tender; Acute posterior lymphadenitis - acute otitis media, and mastoiditis? Various scalp lesions?

- *Tonsillar nodes* – Notable swelling and tenderness in acute tonsillitis? Pharyngitis?

- *Occipital nodes* – Scalp infections? German measles? Roseola infantum?

- *Post auricular* – German measles?

- *Pre-auricular* nodes– Chronic conjunctivitis? Blepharitis? Bacterial infections of same cheek and temporal scalp? Cat-scratch fever?

- *Submandibular nodes* – Infections of the tongue, teeth, gums, lips and cheek.

- *Submental nodes*– Infections of the tip of the tongue and lower lip.

EXAMINATION OF THE AXILLARY NODES
(See Bates p. 464 for position of axillary nodes)

Axillary nodes drain the breast and pleura.

Have the patient relax and support their forearm with your (left) hand. Using firm, gentle, deliberate touch, palpate for lymphadenopathy with the right hand (if you are right handed) at:

- *Central nodes* – High in the apex of axilla.

- *Pectoral nodes* – Grasp the anterior axillary fold with thumb and fingers and palpate inside the border of the pectoral muscle.

- *Lateral nodes* – High in the axilla, along the upper humerus.

- *Subscapular nodes* – From behind the patient, feel inside the muscle of the posterior axillary fold.

Nodes <0.5cm are often palpable in the axilla, but nodes >1cm are nearly always pathological - metastasis cannot be ruled out.

EXAMINATION OF THE INGUINAL NODES
(See Bates p.465 for position of inguinal nodes)

To examine, have the patient lie supine with the knee slightly flexed.

- *Horizontal group* – Inferior to the inguinal ligament.

- *Vertical group* – Inferior to the inguinal ligament, lateral to the genitals and along the line of the femoral vein.

Non-tender, discrete inguinal nodes up to 2cm are frequently palpable in normal people.

SOME LYMPHATIC TERMINOLOGY / PATHOLOGY

Lymphadenopathy refers to enlargement of lymph nodes, with or without tenderness. Try to distinguish between localised (causative lesion in drainage area) and generalised (enlarged nodes in at least two other non-contiguous regions).

Lymphadenitis refers to inflammation of lymph nodes, which become swollen painful and tender.

Lymphangitis refers to inflammation of the lymphatic vessels, seen most commonly as red streaks.

Causes of generalised lymphadenopathy are lymphoma, acute lymphocytic leukaemia (ALL) and chronic lymphocytic leukaemia (CLL), viruses (infective mononucleosis, HIV etc.), bacteria (TB, syphilis), toxoplasmosis (parasitic infection found in cat faeces etc.), and sarcoidosis (granulomatous disease of unknown aetiology).

Causes of localised lymphadenopathy are acute or chronic infection and metastatic cancer.

5. <u>CARDIOVASCULAR EXAMINATION</u>
(See Bates: Chapter 9)

Cardiology is a complex and specialist area but as Herbalists you will be presented with a variety of conditions in some way related to the cardiovascular system. It is important to have a general understanding of the cardiovascular system and related pathologies and to be familiar with key signs and symptoms. The following is meant to provide a comprehensive (but not definitive) check list of signs and symptoms with suggested associated pathologies.

To aid your understanding you should study the pathologies and try to determine why the signs and symptoms occur. Below, for simplicity, a bulleted sign or symptom is commonly followed by associated abnormalities

Patient position to aid examination

- Except for special manoeuvres, cardiac examination should be carried out with the patient supine and the head of the bed raised about 45°

- To establish the apex beat (if undetectable supine) turn the patient to the **left lateral decubitus position** (lay on left side).

- To accentuate aortic murmurs or the soft murmur of aortic insufficiency lean the patient forward.

<u>INSPECTION</u>

GENERAL STATE

- **Pallor** – Fatigue? Fright or general malaise? Shock? Anaemia?

- **Anxiety** – Thyrotoxicosis? Phaeochromocytoma? Psychogenic?

- **Sweating** – Cold sweat of myocardial infarction (MI)? Thyrotoxicosis (hot sweat)? Anxiety (cold sweat)?

- **Peripheral cyanosis** (Blue fingers but pink tongue) – Poor peripheral circulation?

- **Acute dyspnoea** – MI? Left ventricular (LV) failure? Pulmonary embolism? Acute respiratory disease?

- **Chronic dyspnoea** – Cor pulmonale? Chronic obstructive pulmonary disease (COPD)?

- **Orthopnoea** – Sign of LV failure? COPD?

- **Abnormal structure** - Might mimic cardiac pathologies e.g. pectus excavatum or kyphoscoliosis, might cause systolic ejection murmur

HANDS

- **Finger clubbing** – Cyanotic congenital heart disease? Infective endocarditis? RS/GI causes?

- **Blanching of nail beds** (Poor return of colour) – Anaemia?

- **Blanching of palmar creases** (Poor return of colour) – Anaemia?

- **Koilonychia** (Spooning of nails) – Anaemia?

- **Splinter haemorrhages** (Subungual linear haemorrhages) – Infective endocarditis? Trauma?

- **Oslers nodes** (Hard, painful, tender, subcutaneous swelling in fingers toes palms and soles) – Infective endocarditis.

- **Janeway lesions** (Small, flat erythematous non-tender macules on thenar and hypothenar eminence) – Infective endocarditis.

- **Rheumatoid deformities** – Consider cardiac involvement, such as pericarditis or cardiomyopathy.

- **Xanthomas** (on tendons) – Hyperlipidaemia.

- **Capillary pulsation in nailbeds** (Quincke's sign) – Aortic regurgitation.

- **Sclerodactyl** (Finger tapering due to attachment to underlying skin) - Consider systemic sclerosis of heart.

- **Hot and clammy** – Hyperthyroidism?

- **Cold and clammy** – SNS activity, i.e. stress / anxiety?

FACE

- **Pale conjunctiva** – Anaemia (Normally, the anterior portion of the conjunctiva is brighter red than the posterior; in anaemia, this distinction is lost).

- **Bluish discolouration of cheeks** – Mitral facies (face-ease), aka. malar flush - rosy cheeks with bluish tinge. Found in mitral stenosis and is due to dilation of capillaries secondary to pulmonary hypertension.

- **Peaches and cream complexion and fullness of face** – Myxoedema (due to underactive thyroid).

- **High colour of face, sometimes with suffusion of conjunctiva** – Polycythaemia.

- **Tongue** – Blue = central cyanosis (A grave sign - emergency!); Swollen/red (Glossitis) - anaemia?

- **Typical downs syndrome appearance** – Consider atrial septal defect (ASD).

- **Head nodding** (De Musset's sign) – Aortic regurgitation.

- **Xanthelasma** – Hyperlipidaemia.

- **Corneal arcus** (Grey ring on the outer margin of the iris) – Hyperlipidaemia.

- **Argyll Robertson pupils** (Small pupils, react to near effort but not light) – Tertiary syphilis, which is associated with aortic regurgitation, etc.

- **Raised JVP** – Right heart failure? Tricuspid regurgitation? Superior vena cava (SVC) obstruction? (*If you wish to study further, see Chapter 5.1*).

- **Abnormally low JVP** (Cannot be measured so need to lie patient flat to visualise) – Haemorrhage or other forms of hypovolaemia?

- **Goitre** – Thyrotoxicosis (Beware high output heart failure)? Myxoedema (Beware ischaemic heart disease)?

PALPATION

PERIPHERAL PULSES

Examination of arterial pulses enables assessment of heart rate and rhythm, volume and character of the pulse, and assists in detection of blood flow obstruction (see Appendix 1).

Use the pads of the index and middle fingers (or the thumb on larger pulses). If the rhythm is regular count the rate for 15 seconds and multiply by 4. If unusually fast or slow, assess for 60 seconds (This short period is of course for orthodox-style diagnosis).

Know the location of important peripheral pulses, e.g. brachial, radial, radial, temporal etc. (See Appendix 1).

Normal **pulse rate** should be between 60 and 80 BPM, the **rhythm** should be regular (except for obvious sinus-arrhythmia in some young people) and the **character** should be smooth and rounded.

ESTIMATING BLOOD PRESSURE (BP)

It is convenient when testing the pulse to then estimate BP.

The contraction pressure created by the heart is known as systolic and the relaxation pressure is known as diastolic.

The pressures can be measured using a mercury or aneroid sphygmomanometer, or an electronic BP monitor

- Using an appropriate sized cuff, inflate to 30mmHg above the palpable estimated systolic pressure to ensure complete occlusion of the artery. Electronic monitors will usually do the rest.

- If using an aneroid or mercury sphygmomanometer, listen for the (Korotkoff) sounds of the pulse with a stethoscope placed over the brachial artery, the cuff is gradually deflated.

- The pressure at which the pulse is first heard in the artery is the systolic pressure.

- The cuff continues to be deflated, and at some point, the sound of blood flowing stops and this is the diastolic pressure. Record both sounds (see Appendix 2)

PALPATION OF ANTERIOR CHEST (praecordium)

- **Apex beat / left ventricular heaves** Normally palpable around 4th or 5th intercostal space at or just medial to mid-clavicular line (normal apex is impalpable in 50%)

  - **Visible** – Hyperdynamic states? Thin patient?

  - **Shifted** – Inferior and lateral shift could mean cardiac enlargement?

  - **Heaving, sustained** – Left ventricular hypertrophy due to hypertension?

- o **Impulse on right** – Dexterocardia? Right ventricular hypertrophy?

- o **Thrusting** (i.e. Heaving, not sustained) – Volume overload e.g. mitral/aortic regurgitation?

- o **Tapping** – Mitral stenosis (Palpable first heart sound)?

- o **Double impulse** – Dyskinetic or aneurismal segment of left ventricle? Hypertrophic obstructive cardiomyopathy (Hypertrophy causes forceful atrial contraction)?

- o **Absent impulse** – Obesity? Emphysema? Pericardial effusion? (By inhibition of sound transmission).

- **Right ventricular heaves** palpable at lower left lateral sternal border – right heart failure (Might be left atrial hypertrophy)?

- **Abnormal impulse** palpable at left 2nd intercostal space - Severe pulmonary hypertension?

- **Abnormal impulse** palpable at right 2nd intercostal space – upper aortic aneurism?

- **Thrills** (Palpable loud murmurs) – definite abnormality e.g. stenotic or incompetent valves?

ABDOMINAL SIGNS

- **Ascites** – Severe congestive heart failure (CHF)? Constrictive pericarditis? Liver disease?

- **Expansile aortic pulsation** – Aortic aneurism.

- **Hepatomegaly** (on palpation) – CHF (Smooth and rounded)? Tricuspid regurgitation (Pulsatile)? Liver disease (Hard with irregular edge)?

- **Renal Artery Bruits** (on auscultation) – Renal artery stenosis (Curable form of hypertension).

Oedema is a common symptom and sign of heart failure (Also occurs in many other situations) – caused by increased venous pressure, and fluid overload related to changes in renal blood flow resulting in sodium and water retention.

- **Pitting oedema** – persistent indentation caused by pressing for 5 seconds (e.g. around medial aspect of the lower shin). This occurs because subcutaneous tissues are filled with low protein fluid (as in heart failure)

- **Non-pitting oedema** – caused by proteinaceous fluid (e.g. due to lymphatic obstruction by tumour). In the early stages pitting occurs (After pressing for 30 seconds). Later, the oedematous area fibroses and hardens giving a brawny appearance. Pitting then no longer occurs

AUSCULTATION

NORMAL HEART SOUNDS

A complete knowledge of cardiac auscultation is a specialist technique that requires prolonged practice in a clinical setting.

Proficiency requires a sound knowledge and recognition of normal heart sounds so that when abnormal sounds occur you will recognise them and refer if necessary.

The diaphragm of the stethoscope pressed firmly on the chest is used to listen to higher frequency sounds such as that of mitral valve closure (S1).

The bell held lightly is used to listen to lower frequency sounds such as S3 and S4

- S_1 (*Lub*) - closure of mitral valve or tricuspid valve

- o Caused by initiation of ventricular contraction.

- o Heard at apex (Mitral) and LLSB (Tricuspid) with diaphragm of stethoscope.

- **S₂ (*Dup*)** - closure of aortic valve or pulmonic valve

  - o Occurs when left ventricular pressure is lower than aortic pressure (end of systole).

  - o Heard at base right (Aortic) and base left (Pulmonic) with diaphragm of stethoscope.

IDENTIFYING THE TIMING OF S1 AND S2

To identify these paired sounds, know that there is a relatively long diastolic interval.

S1 is usually louder (indicated by the longer line in the diagram) than S2 at the apex; S2 is usually louder than S1 at the base e.g.

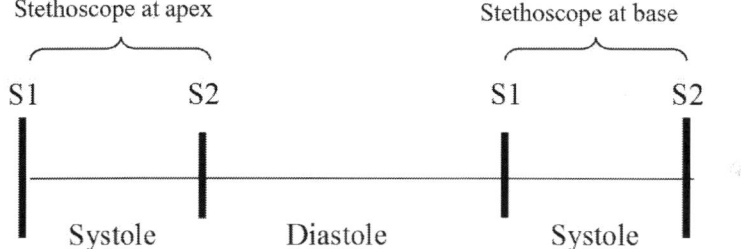

DETECTING AN ABNORMALITY

How easy it is to detect an abnormality depends on the abnormality. Firstly, you should positively identify and decide if S1 and S2 are normal.

- S1 might be increased in tachycardia, mitral stenosis and high output states such as anaemia, hyperthyroidism and exercise.

- S1 might be decreased in first degree heart block, a calcified valve as found with mitral regurgitation, and when ventricular contractility is reduced as in CHF

- S2 might be decreased in aortic stenosis

Next, you should decide if the abnormality is a "bump" or a murmur (Try to access credible audio recordings of normal and abnormal heart sounds).

AUSCULTATE LUNG BASES

Crackles are an early sign of pulmonary oedema and CHF

5.1 <u>ESTIMATION OF JUGULAR VENOUS PRESSURE (JVP)</u>
(Not useful under 12 years – unable to detect)

<u>GENERAL</u>
(See Bates: pp. 299-301)

The venous pulse can be assessed more readily on the right than on the left side of the neck, because the right brachiocephalic and jugular veins extend in an almost straight line to the superior vena cava, favouring transmission of the haemodynamic changes from the right atrium (see diagram below).

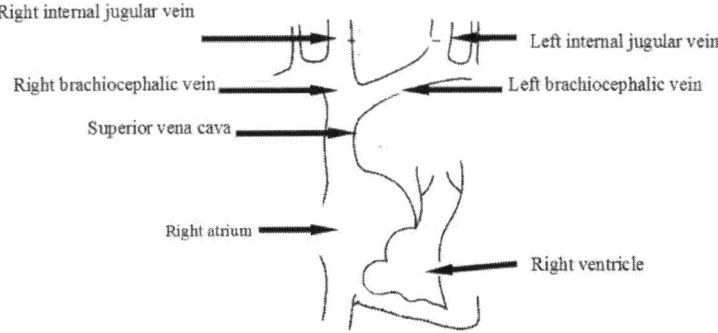

The soft, rapid, double pulsation of the internal jugular veins represents the changing pressure within the right atrium, it is useful to understand the causes.

Cause of the double pulsation of JVP:

A wave: Back pressure from atrial contraction (Precedes S1).

X descent: Pulling down from right ventricular contraction.

V wave: Atrial filling – atrial pressure begins to rise (Almost coincides with S2).

Y descent: Tricuspid opening.

There are thought to be no valves between the internal jugular vein and the right atrium, therefore observation of the column of blood in it enables a reasonably reliable estimation of right atrial pressure.

METHOD OF ESTIMATING JVP

- Position the patient at 45° with their head tilted slightly away from the side you are observing and slightly flexed (elicits a relaxed sternomastoid).

- In a normal person, JVP might be detectable but not normally rising above the clavicle (between the origins of the sternomastoid on the sternum and clavicle).

- The above method is suitable for our purposes but elevations can be measured (Those greater than 3 or 4cm above the sternal angle are considered elevated).

How to distinguish JVP pulsation from carotid pulsation

JVP	Carotid
Normally not palpable	Palpable
Soft, rapid, double elevation/ heart beat	Vigorous, single elevation
Eliminated by pressure	Not eliminated by pressure
Level of pulsation changes with position	Level of pulsation unchanged by position
Usually descends with inspiration	Level not affected by inspiration

ABNORMAL JVP INDICATIONS

- **Raised JVP** – Right heart failure (Most common cause of raised JVP) usually secondary to left heart failure caused by ischaemic heart disease or mitral valve disease. May be secondary to pulmonary disease (Cor pulmonale).

- **Raised JVP** – Fluid overload as in kidney failure or excess intravenous fluids.

- **Raised JVP** (distended and non-pulsatile) - SVC obstruction usually due to mediastinal lymphadenopathy secondary to lung cancer.

- **Raised JVP** (large V with slow descent) – Tricuspid regurgitation.

- **Raised JVP** (large "cannon" A) – Tricuspid stenosis, pulmonic stenosis, pulmonary hypertension, complete heart block.

- **Raised JVP** (with absent A) – Atrial fibrillation ∴ no atrial systole ∴ no A wave.

- **Abnormally low JVP** (i.e. cannot be measured - need to lie patient flat) – Haemorrhage or other forms of hypovolaemia.

- **Raised JVP** (on inspiration, deep Y descent) – Constrictive pericarditis.

Notes

If JVP is extremely elevated, the top of the pulsation may be above the neck and so not visible. In this case the patient should be sat upright.

The internal jugular vein can be very difficult to examine; it takes lots of practice. However, persevere because it is an important indicator of cardiac and pulmonary disease.

5.2 OPTHALMOSCOPY – CARDIOVASCULAR

Ophthalmoscopy is a specialist technique so do not become disheartened when unable to locate structures but do not expect to become proficient without practice.

EXAMINATION METHOD

Darken the room, switch on the ophthalmoscope, set it to the large or medium round beam (Some authorities suggest starting with a small beam but use this if the pupil is constricted), and 0 diopters*

A diopter is a unit that measures the power of the lens to converge/diverge light. Adjust this as necessary. An optician might adjust this in relation to their own and the patient's prescription.

To examine the fundus of the patient's right eye:
(See Bates: Table 7.9)

Hold the ophthalmoscope in the **right** hand and up to your **right** eye to examine the patient's **right** eye, i.e. **right, right, right.** (Left, left, left for examining left eye).

1. With the patient seated, stand at the patient's right side about $15 - 25^{o.}$

2. Ask the patient to fix their gaze at a given point ahead and slightly up.

3. Position the ophthalmoscope 15 inches (38cm) from the patient.

4. Rest your left hand on the patient's forehead with the thumb on the eyebrow (assists proprioceptive guidance).

5. Direct the light-beam onto the patient's pupil, a red reflex should appear (like a flash photo). An opaque lens will inhibit this (e.g. as in cataracts or detached retina).

6. With the patient's gaze fixed, slowly move toward the patient keeping the reflex in view.

7. At approximately 1½ - 2 inches (4-5cm) you should (with practice) see the optic disc – a yellow/orange to creamy pink oval or round structure where the blood vessels converge.

Tips for use

- If either you or the patient is **myopic** (can see near but not far – light rays focus anterior to retina), focus the instrument by resetting the diopters, i.e. rotate the dial counter-clockwise, from 0 through the minus or red numbers.

- If either you or the patient is **hyoperopic** (can see far but not near – light rays focus posterior to retina) then rotate the diopters clockwise, from 0 through the plus or green numbers.

- Unless you have marked myopia or severe astigmatism remove your glasses, likewise the patient. There is no need for you or the patient to remove contact lenses.

EXAMINE FOR HYPERTENSIVE RETINOPATHY
(See Bates: Table 7.10 – 7.14)

Assessing retinal arteries is in a sense assessing all arteries. Hypertension damages vessels of the retina, the level being dependent on severity. Grading indicates severity (Grade 4 being malignant hypertension). Authorities tend to vary with regard to some aspects of grading but the following is generally useful in identifying hypertensive retinopathy:

- **Normal** – Light reflex in arteries (only).

- **Grade 1** – Arterial narrowing in relation to veins, vessels become tortuous. Arteries (nearer to the disc) may become tortuous (Particularly due to arteriosclerosis. Tortuous retinal veins are also associated with hypertension, but in particular, when associated with occlusion of the central retinal vein). Copper or silver wiring may be seen.

- **Grade 2** – All above plus AV nipping

- **Grade 3** - All above plus haemorrhages and cotton wool exudates.

- **Grade 4** – All above plus papilloedema (Disc margin blurs outward).

6. RESPIRATORY EXAMINATION
(See Bates: Chapter 8)

GENERAL

- Examination of the posterior chest is best done with the patient sitting forward with arms crossed at the chest, to separate the scapula and make the lung fields more accessible.

- The anterior chest may also be examined with the patient sitting but is more readily accessible, particularly the female anterior thorax, with the patient at 45^0 or supine.

- You should examine the bare chest and back where possible, explain that you can cover the chest with a sheet during examination but give the patient the opportunity to refuse.

- If the patient's thorax is particularly hairy it might be necessary to press the diaphragm firmer or wet the hair to reduce rustling, which may mask other sounds.

The general routine should be **Inspection - Palpation - Percussion – Auscultation.** For ease of learning in anatomical sequence and to ensure complete examination some palpation has been included in inspection.

INSPECTION

HANDS
- **Finger clubbing** – Bronchiectasis? Bronchial carcinoma? Lung abscess? Empyema (pus in pleural cavity)? Fibrosing alveolitis? COPD (some authorities dispute this connection)? Cardiovascular or GIT diseases?

- **Cyanosis** – Might be peripheral but suspect central, i.e. COPD and heart disease

- **Blanching of nail beds and palmar creases** – Anaemia?

- **Bounding pulse** – Hypercapnia (increased CO_2)? Anaemia? Asthma (>110 BPM is severe attack; If accompanied by bradycardia, this is life-threatening cardiac insufficiency)? Chest infection/pneumonia?

- **Flapping tremor** – Hypercapnia?

FACE

- **Central cyanosis** – COPD? Heart disease?

- **Moon face** – Steroid therapy? Cushing's syndrome?

- **Horner's syndrome** – Apical carcinoma encroaching on cervical sympathetic chain. Results in hemifacial pupillary constriction, partial ptosis and anhidrosis (loss of sweating).

- **Pale conjunctiva** – Anaemia (the anterior is normally brighter red compared to the posterior)?

- **Sinus tenderness** (Press up under frontal and maxillary sinuses to elicit tenderness) – Sinusitis?

- **Pursed lip breathing** – Emphysema?

- **Audible sounds** – *Wheeze*, *stridor* (inspirational high pitched noise). If accompanied by a barking cough, consider **Croup**. If accompanied by a paroxysmal cough followed by inspiratory whoop (in 50%) consider **Whooping cough**?

- **Grunting** (Healthy babies may grunt to defecate or show happiness) in a sickly baby grunting is a serious sign (Medical emergency). Grunting with exhalation and rapid shallow breathing indicates lower respiratory tract infection - May represent pneumonia, asthma, bronchiolitis, meningitis or heart failure.

NECK

- **JVP** – Raised in cor pulmonale. (at 45^0 angle, should normally not see or only just see pulsation)

- **Tracheal deviation** – Mediastinal displacement by collapse or fibrosis pulls the trachea to the side of the lesion; Deviation caused by effusion, pneumothorax or tumour pushes the trachea from the side of the lesion. (If deviation is found, the apex beat may also be assessed at this time to confirm mediastinal shift)

- **Crico-sternal distance** (normally a 2 finger distance between the cricoid cartilage and suprasternal notch) - Reduced in emphysema and asthma.

- **Palpate for lymphadenopathy** – Neoplasia or infection.

  - *Supraclavicular* – Important when suspecting intra-abdominal or intra-thoracic structure. Tumours may metastasise to these nodes.

  - *Cervical nodes* – Viral URT infections usually non-tender. Glandular fever - may be quite tender. Acute posterior lymphadenitis in acute otitis media and mastoiditis and various scalp lesions.

  - *Tonsillar nodes* – Notable swelling and tenderness in acute tonsillitis; Pharyngitis?

  - *Occipital nodes* – Scalp infections? German measles? Roseola infantum?

  - *Pre-auricular nodes*– Chronic conjunctivitis? Blepharitis? Bacterial infections of same cheek and temporal scalp? Cat-scratch fever?

  - *Submandibular nodes* – Infections of the tongue, teeth, gums, lips and cheek.

  - *Submental nodes*– Infections of the tip of the tongue and lower lip.

- **Supraclavicular retraction and use of breathing accessory muscles** – Severe difficulty in breathing as in COPD and asthma.

- **Assess breathing rate** – Normal adults, 14-20/min; new-born, 30-60/min; early childhood, 20-40/min.

- **Tachypnoea** – Anxiety? Hypercapnea and hypoxia as in asthma/COPD? Pneumonia? Pulmonary embolism? Pleuritic chest pain? Heart disease?

- **Bradypnoea** – Opiate overdose? Neurological conditions such as stroke or raised intracranial pressure (ICP)?

- **Abnormal retraction of costal interspaces** – Severe asthma? COPD?

- **Kyphoscoliosis** – Can interfere with inspiration (i.e. a restrictive lung disease)

PALPATION

- **Assess chest expansion** (Front and back)

    o **Normal** - Should be at least 5cm separation (between examiner's thumbs on inhalation) and symmetrical.

    o **Diminished** – Consolidation? Atelectasis? Fibrosis? Pneumothorax? Large effusion? Lung abscess? etc. (Pathology on side of diminished expansion, also rises on inspiration).

- **Assess Tactile Vocal Fremitus** (Front and back) Most effective in evaluating areas found dull to percussion. Most physicians prefer vocal resonance.

    o **Increased TVF** – Consolidation?

    o **Decreased TVF** – Effusion or collapse?

- **Tenderness** – Intercostal tenderness of inflamed pleura or an exquisitely painful area might suggest rib fracture (associated crepitus).

PERCUSSION (Front, back and side)

Percuss at the midpoint of your middle finger of the left hand (Pleximeter) with the pad of the middle finger of the right (Plexor). The right hand remains firm, allowing gravity to assist wrist flexion.

- **Resonance** – Normal.

- **Dullness** – Consolidation (alveoli filled with fluid from inflamed lungs e.g. pneumonia)? Fibrosis? Collapse? Tumour? Liver/heart/spleen/lymph?

- **Stony dull** – Pleural effusion?

- **Hyper-resonance** – Over-inflation? Emphysema? Pneumothorax?

AUSCULTATION (Front, back and side)

Lung sounds are generally low pitched and therefore, some sources recommend using the bell of the stethoscope. However, it is common to use the diaphragm. Alternatively, use the bell for low-pitched sounds and the diaphragm for high pitched, e.g. aegophony. Cover the same areas as percussion, if you hear a problem, examine the area more fully.

BREATH SOUNDS

- **Vesicular** – Normal.

- **Bronchial** (over trachea) – Normal.

- **Bronchial** (other than at the trachea and possibly right apex) - Alveolar damage as in consolidation, collapse or fibrosis.

- **Diminished vesicular** – Collapse? Fibrosis? COPD? Also, might be found in obese, muscular or elderly?

- **Absent** – Large pleural effusion? Massive atelectasis (failure of lung or part of lung to expand)?

- **Crackles** (aka. Rales) – Early CHF? Pulmonary oedema? Pneumonia? Bronchitis? Bronchiectasis?

- **Wheezes** – Due to narrowed airways, e.g. Asthma? COPD? Bronchitis? Tumour? Foreign body?

- **Rhonchi** – Due to large airway secretion, e.g. Pneumonia? Chronic bronchitis? Bed–ridden or post-operative patient?

- **Stridor** (inspiratory wheeze, often audible) – Obstruction of larynx or trachea.

- **Pleural friction rub** – Pleural inflammation (pleurisy).

<u>VOCAL RESONANCE</u> (Front and back)

- **Bronchophony** (patient says "99") and **Whispered Pectoriloquay** (patient whispers 99).

  - **Increased** – Consolidation?

  - **Decreased** – Pleural effusion or collapse?

- **Aegophony** (patient says "E") – sounds like "A" in consolidation and at the upper border of pleural effusion.

HOW RS SIGNS CAN ADD UP IN DISEASE STATES

To assist learning and practice the above findings are given separately, actuality, signs and symptoms usually "add up". For example, if you find bronchial breathing over the parenchyma, you will also find increased TVF, VR etc. If this is not the case, then you probably not have heard bronchial sounds. Here are some examples of respiratory pathology and associated signs:

- **Consolidation** – Area of lung filled with fluid or solid matter – classically **infective pneumonia** which affects enough lung to give also reduced expansion, dull percussion, increased TVF and VR and bronchial breathing.

  Consolidation is also a feature of **pulmonary haemorrhage** and **pneumonitis** (Inflammation due to non-infective causes, e.g. drugs, autoimmune). In these conditions, signs are variable.

- **Pleural effusion** – Abnormal amount of serous fluid in the pleural space resulting in reduced expansion, stony-dull percussion, reduced TVF and VR, reduced/commonly absent vesicular breathing and tracheal and apical displacement away from effusion (if effusion is large).

  Pleural effusion is due to such conditions as pneumonia, tumours, TB (Exudates – high protein content); or heart failure, hypoalbuminaemia, pulmonary emboli (Transudates – low protein content).

  Other types of fluid in pleural space may be due to **haemothorax** (blood), **chylothorax** (Chyle), **empyema** (Pus)

- **Lung collapse** – Due to a blocked bronchus, the air in the lung distal to the blockage is reabsorbed leaving a partially collapsed lung. This results in reduced expansion, dull percussion, reduced TVF and VR, reduced vesicular breathing but may be any area of bronchial breathing and tracheal deviation toward the area, if large.

- **Pneumothorax** – Air in pleural space due to leakage from the lung through the visceral pleura – loss of negative pressure in space therefore, loss of maintained inflation and collapse. This results in <u>reduced</u> expansion, hyper-resonant percussion, reduced TVF and VR, reduced vesicular breathing. Pneumothorax can be spontaneous or due to trauma.

See also lymph node examination, ear examination and examination of oral cavity for relevant respiratory tract examination, signs and symptoms.

7. ABDOMINAL EXAMINATION
(See Bates: Chapter 11)

GENERAL

Explain to the patient that you wish to carry out an abdominal examination (e.g. "Do you mind if I examine your hands and tummy") and if they approve assist them onto the couch. To elicit a relaxed abdomen, it is sometimes useful to place a pillow under the patient's knees as well as their head (NB an arched back cause tightening of the abdominal muscles).

First, inspect the patient's hands and face (be considerate and gentle but look and feel like you know what you are doing). Following on, ask them to expose their abdomen, always being concerned for their modesty. Before you palpate and percuss, explain to the patient what you are going to do and encourage them to let you know if something is uncomfortable, tender or painful. Of course, as you examine the patient you will be observing their facial expression and feeling for guarding.

When palpating, do not dig and poke, use careful, firm pressure with rhythmic movements. Work from the patient's right side and visualise each organ in the region you are examining.

INSPECTION

HANDS

- **Finger clubbing** – Inflammatory bowel disease? Chronic liver disease? Non-gut causes?

- **Leukonychia** (white on nails) – Trauma? Cirrhosis of the liver? Nephritic syndrome?

- **Koilonychia** ('spooning') – Due to chronic iron deficiency: GI bleeding from ulcer or tumour? Malnutrition? Worms? Coelic?

- **Liver palm** (palmar erythema) - Chronic liver disease?

- **Palmer fibromatosis** (Dupuytren's contracture) – Chronic liver disease? Alcoholic cirrhosis?

- **Xanthomas** (in palmar creases) – Primary biliary cirrhosis?

- **Flapping tremor** (patient extends arms, cocks the hand back at the wrists and spreads fingers – expect twitch downwards) – Liver failure?

FACE/MOUTH

- **Cachexia** – Suggests malignancy.

- **Sallow complexion** (unhealthy looking, lustreless, lack of vitality) – Renal failure? Anaemia? Vitamin B deficiency?

- **Rhynophyma** – Acne rosacea, a complication in alcoholics - may have cirrhosis

- **Parotid swelling** – Stones? Infection? Tumour?

- **Yellow sclerae** – Increased bilirubin.

- **Xanthelasma** – Hyperlipidaemia, if jaundiced consider primary biliary cirrhosis.

- **Pallor** – Anaemia?

- **Conjunctival pallor** -Anaemia?

- **Angular stomatitis** – Anaemia?

- **Inflamed/sore tongue** – Anaemia?

- **Apthous ulcers** – Increased risk of UC in some people? Painless ulcer may be beginning of squamous carcinoma?

- **Breath odour** – Sweet, musty smell – liver failure? Acetone (pear drops) – diabetic ketoacidosis, alcohol? Foul-smelling (halitosis) – poor dental hygiene? Pathology of nasopharynx? Bronchiectasis?

- **Scratch marks** (from itching) – Increased bilirubin?

- **Yellow discolouration** – Increased bilirubin?

- **Bruises** – Chronic liver disease (clotting deficiency)? Blood disease?

- **Tattoos/piercing** – Association with Hepatitis B.

- **Spider naevi** – Chronic liver disease? - (>6 in distribution of the SVC and almost never below the waist). Also, found in pregnancy and B vitamin deficiency. Sometimes occur in healthy people.

- **Dermatitis herpetiformis** – Coeliac disease?

ABDOMEN

- **Very thin** – Starvation? Malabsorption? Wasting disease?

- **Ascites** (fluid) – Cirrhosis, associated with portal hypertension and hypoalbuminaemia? Malignancy? CHF? Nephrotic syndrome?

- **Distension other than ascites** – Fat? Faeces? Flatus? Foetus? Tumour?

- **Abdominal striae** – Previous pregnancy? Obesity? Cushing's syndrome (purple)?

- **Scars** – Previous surgery?

- **Distended abdominal veins** – Radiating from umbilicus (caput medusae) - suggests portal hypertension? Coursing vertically - suggests inferior vena cava obstruction?

- **Asymmetry of abdomen** - Due to an enlarged organ or mass?

- **Abnormal pulsation** – Aortic aneurysm?

- **Visible peristalsis** – Obstruction?

- **Abdomen held rigid** – Peritonitis?

- **Lump in femoral region** – Hernia?

AUSCULTATION

In contrast to examination of the CVS and RS, some authorities suggest auscultation prior to palpation and percussion, as these may alter frequency of bowel sounds. In addition, others suggest auscultation may only be appropriate if there are other abnormal findings. However, if the case history suggests bowel obstruction you should auscultate prior to palpation, because it is suggested that in some cases, palpation might provoke a paralytic ileus. If auscultation indicates obstruction and the patient demonstrates guarding when you touch them, you should abandon the examination and immediately refer.

Normal sounds consist of clicks and gurgles occurring at a frequency of 5 to 34 per minute. Listening in only one spot is usually sufficient, i.e. right lower quadrant. Listen for at least 30 seconds, but before deciding bowel sounds are absent, listen for 2 minutes.

- **Bowel sounds**

  o Diminished or absent suggests paralytic ileus.

  o Tinkling high pitched sounds-intestinal obstruction.

Note: Four main symptoms of acute obstruction are colicky pain, distension, faeculent vomiting and absolute constipation even to flatus.

- **Bruits**

  o **Renal artery bruits** (auscultate over renal arteries)– Renal artery stenosis?

- ○ **Hepatic bruits** (auscultate over liver around right costal margin) – Carcinoma of liver? Alcoholic cirrhosis?

PALPATION
(With warm hands and short fingernails)

GENERAL PALPATION
For light palpation use one hand, for deep palpation use two hands. With deep palpation, the hand in contact with the abdomen should be used as a sensor only, the upper hand is used to apply deeper pressure and movement.

Palpate for intra-abdominal masses assessing: size, shape, number, tenderness, mobility, temperature, colour of underlying skin, relation to surrounding tissue, pulsation, sounds on auscultation. (See causes of abdominal masses below)

Asking the patient to take a deep breath and relax as they breathe out through an open mouth will allow more sensitive and deeper palpation. **NB. If rigidity persists despite this technique the guarding may be involuntary and indicates peritoneal inflammation, immediately refer.**

- • **Rebound tenderness** – Suggests peritoneal inflammation.

- • **Pain on coughing** – Suggests peritoneal inflammation.

Tip

To distinguish an intra-abdominal mass from a mass in the abdominal wall, ask patient to raise head and shoulders to tighten the abdominal muscles; an intra-abdominal mass will be obscured by the contraction. (See table below showing some cause of abdominal mass)

Assess liver borders
Unlike assessing the abdomen, palpate deeply as the patient inhales.

Normally, the lower border may or may not be palpable below the right costal margin.

NB. The upper border must be determined by percussion to differentiate between an enlarged or a displaced liver.

- **Hepatomegaly**

  o Hard, irregular, non-tender - Cancer (probably metastatic)?

  o Smooth, firm, non-tender - Lymphoma? Early cirrhosis?

  o Smooth, tender - Infection? CHF?

- **Tenderness in a non-palpable liver** - Infection as in hepatitis? Congestion as in heart failure?

GALL BLADDER PALPATION

- **Rebound tenderness** – Suggests peritonitis.

- **Murphy's sign** – Cholecystitis. (Hook thumb or fingers under costal margin around R9 or under liver edge if enlarged - increased tenderness and inspiratory arrest is a positive Murphy's sign).

SPLEEN PALPATION (on inspiration)

- **<u>NB. This is a potentially dangerous technique that might cause rupture!</u>** – If unsure whether to palpate, **percuss** the lowest intercostal interspace at left anterior axillary line – there is normally a tympanic response. Ask patient to take a deep breath and percuss again. If normal it should remain tympanic

- **Splenomegaly** – Infection? Portal hypertension? Blood disorders?

NB. If splenomegaly is suspected, begin palpation in right iliac fossa otherwise the lower border may not be detected.

KIDNEY PALPATION (on inspiration)

- **Enlargement**- Tumour? Polycystic disease? Hydronephrosis?

- **Tenderness** – Suggests infection.

ADDITIONAL ABDOMINAL TESTS
(For suspected appendicitis)

- **Ask patient to cough** – Pain increases due to increased intra-abdominal pressure on the inflammation.

- **Tenderness on palpation in RIF** and surrounding areas (even the right flank).

- **Early guarding** leading to rigidity later.

- **Rebound tenderness** (pain on removal of pressure**) at McBurney's point** – Due to peritoneal inflammation (Avoid if other signs are positive).

- **Rovsing's sign** – Pain in RIF with pressure in LIF (also, referred rebound tenderness).

- **Psoas sign** – Ask the patient to flex their knee against your resistance – abdominal pain suggests irritation of psoas muscle by inflamed appendix. Also, on passive hip extension in the left lateral decubitus position

- **Obturator sign** – Flex the patient's right hip, bend knee and rotate internally at the hip (Stretches the obturator muscle) – hypogastric pain suggests irritation of obturator muscle by inflamed appendix.

- **Cutaneous hyperaesthesia** – Gently pick up folds of skin along the abdominal wall (without pinching) – localised pain in RIF may indicate appendicitis.

PERCUSSION

- **Protuberant abdomen, tympanic throughout** – Intestinal obstruction?

- **Large dull areas** – Underlying mass or enlarged organ, e.g. Pregnant uterus? Ovarian tumour? Distended bladder? Enlarged liver or spleen?

- **Pain on percussion** – Peritoneal inflammation?

NB Tympani is usually the result of gas in the GI tract and scattered areas of dullness are typically due to fluid and faeces.

Use percussion to estimate liver borders and spleen size if indicated by other abnormal findings, i.e. during inspection, general percussion and palpation.

EXAMINATION OF HERNIAL ORIFICES AND EXTERNAL GENITALIA

- **Indirect hernia** – Swelling above inguinal ligament often extending into scrotum or labia.

- **Direct hernia** – Swelling above inguinal ligament close to pubic tubercle, rarely into scrotum.

- **Femoral hernia** – Swelling below inguinal ligament, never into scrotum.

If there are no swellings and you suspect a hernia, ask the patient to cough, a consequent bulge suggests an occult hernia. Then place your hand over the swelling and ask the patient to cough while you feel the impulse and identify its nature.

SOME CAUSES OF ABDOMINAL MASS
(Not definitive)
Causes of epigastric mass
Stomach - Cancer, pyloric stenosis
Liver - enlarged left lobe
Pancreatic cyst, cancer in head of pancreas
Gallbladder - Mucocoele / empyaema
Causes of right iliac fossa mass
Caecum - Carcinoma, Crohn's, TB
Appendix - Appendix abscess
Ovary - Cyst, carcinoma
Psoas - Psoas abscess
External iliac artery - Aneurism
Pelvic kidney (fails to reach adult level)
Causes of left iliac fossa mass
Sigmoid colon - Cancer, diverticular abscess
Ovary - Cyst, carcinoma
Psoas - Psoas abscess
External iliac artery - Aneurism
Causes of hypogastric mass
Enlarged bladder, Ovarian cyst, Tumour of sigmoid colon.

8. MUSCULOSKELETAL EXAMINATION
(See Bates: Chapter 17)

EXAMINATION OF THE SPINE

GENERAL

Back pain commonly results from injury through activity. Occasionally back pain may have more sinister causes - be aware of: fever and unexplained weight loss; bladder/bowel dysfunction; history of cancer; progressive neurological deficit; steroid use; HIV infection; disturbed gait or saddle anaesthesia; onset before age 20 or after age 55.

8.1 CERVICAL SPINE

INSPECTION

- Look for signs of pain, stiffness and swelling (Nerve root compression involves paraesthesia and weakness). NB. Pain may also radiate to the limbs, head or back of head resulting also in headache.

- Look for muscle wasting particularly in the upper limbs – thenar/hypothenar eminence and dorsal interosseous muscle (apparent by raised tendons and hollows).

- Look for asymmetry, e.g. swelling – abscesses due to something underlying local musculature or spasms.

PALPATION (Patient sitting)

- Hold the forehead with one hand and palpate with the other for obvious bony or muscular changes, tenderness or spasm.

- Palpate joint capsules.

    o Soft, inflamed and tender – indicates recent acute episode.

- Hard, bony, swollen and not so painful – indicates chronic condition and therefore, fibrotic (Picture becomes complicated when old lesions become acute).

- Identify the level of the problem, i.e. upper? middle? lower? may give a clue to lesion, e.g.

  Upper cervicals – Rheumatoid arthritis?
  Lower cervicals - Osteoarthritis?
  Middle cervicals - Whiplash?

MOBILITY

These tests are mainly for gross mobility in all directions. First carry out active tests then passive tests, and proceed with caution!

Active - Patient sitting. Direct the patient to "keep your shoulders still and move your head only"

- **Flexion** - Direct the patient to move chin to chest with jaw closed. Note limitation in flexion, pain etc. Paraesthesia in the arms and sometimes legs can occur in multiple sclerosis (***Lhermitte's sign***).

- **Extension** – Direct the patient to lean head back to look up. Note limitation, pain etc. Paraesthesia in extension is due to cervical myelopathy (stenosis/spondylosis) i.e. pressure on spinal cord/vessels (***Reverse Lhermitte's sign***).

- **Lateral flexion** – Direct the patient to move ear to shoulder. Compare sides etc.

- **Rotation** – Direct the patient to keep body still and with head only turn from left to right. Note limitation of movement.

  Rotation in flexion tests C1, C2, C3.
  Rotation in neutral tests C4, C5.
  Rotation in extension tests C5, C6, C7

Passive – With the patient supine (or seated) feel for bony, springy movements, crepitus, etc.

- Hold the occiput in one hand and then with the other, carefully move the patient's head to elicit cervical **flexion, extension, lateral flexion** and **rotation**.

- **Cervical compression test** (To reproduce pain/paraesthesia)

    NB This test is potentially dangerous, and should only be carried out under supervision or if experienced - be very careful)

    Inform the patient of your intentions and ask them to inform you if pain/paraesthesia is reproduced. Support the back of the neck and **gently** compress the top of the head. If this does not show anything try the next test.

- If symptom on left, **gently** – flex the neck slightly, rotate to right, side bend to left, then extend. If symptoms on the right, then vice versa.

NB. Pain caused by these techniques may be caused by a disc pathology, spondylosis, tumour or fracture so you should **REFER.**

GOLDEN RULE: UNIVERSAL LIMITATION INDICATES A SERIOUS UNDERLYING PATHOLOGY, E.G. FRACTURE OR TUMOUR.
DO NOT TOUCH OR MOVE THE PERSON! CALL THE PARAMEDICS.

8.2 THE THORACIC AND LUMBOSACRAL SPINE

INSPECTION
(Observe from back and side)

- Look for hyper-lordosis, scoliosis, kyphosis and kyphoscoliosis.

- Look for ordinary pattern, e.g. how the arms hang (look for rotation indication distortion e.g. pelvis).

- Look for unusual muscle tone or atrophy (e.g. erector spinae and antagonist – rectus femorus).

- Look for scars and marks (Café–au-lait patches, skin tags and fibrous tumours in neurofibromatosis – tumours of peripheral nerve covering which may appear in spinal canal and press on spinal cord. Birthmarks, port wine stains, hairy patches and lipomas overlie bony defects such as in spina bifida).

Notes on scoliosis

- To establish whether scoliosis is functional or structural ask patient to sit down or lie prone. Functional scoliosis is caused by pain (most common cause) and will disappear on resting. NB. It is common to have a little scoliosis.

- Be aware of seeing scoliosis in young girls – aetiology is unknown but if not corrected it may develop into a chronic permanent condition.

- Pelvic distortion may cause scoliosis - perhaps a short leg (measure for apparent and true leg length) or fallen arch. So never look at problem in isolation – extreme back pain may be due to a stiff neck!

PALPATION

- Feel muscles for tone.

- Feel and percuss over spine to determine area of tenderness e.g. if pain is over a spinous process, it may be a joint problem (Painful vertebra may be disc collapse, disc infection, tumour); if over the sacroiliac, it may be sacroiliitis.

- Assess level of pelvis – use both thumbs and come under the posterior superior iliac spine (PSIS aka. Dimples of Venus) until you feel it. Look at the level of your thumbs. Are they higher or lower? Is one deeper? Perhaps most common – one ilium rotates forward and other backward.

  If one thumb is deeper and higher, this is a tilted pelvis (perhaps due to a short leg).

MOBILITY

Active (with the patient standing)

- **Flexion** – Patient tucks in chin with arms hanging down and see how far the patient can flex (Persistent lumbar lordosis suggests spasm or ankylosing spondylitis). Looking from behind, a suspected scoliosis can become more visible in this posture.

- **Extension** – Support the patient and ask them to lean back.

- **Lateral flexion** – Standing straight, the patient slides the left hand down the left leg and then the right hand down the right leg (stabilise the pelvis to prevent compensatory movement).

- **Rotation** – Standing straight the patient turns the body left and right (stabilise the pelvis).

Passive (Patient lying down)

In most cases, you may be satisfied with active examination, so there may be no need for passive.

- **Flexion** No specific test (at this level) but may use The straight leg raise (SLR) to establish muscle or root compression (Sciatica)

- **Sacroiliac testing** – With the patient prone (relaxing the erector spinae), press the heel of your palm on the patient's sacroiliac. Alternatively, semi-flex leg and externally rotate hip (lifts the pelvis) and at the same time press down.

- **Lateral flexion** – Patient knee flexion to 90° and use the foot as a lever. Flex laterally and use thumb and finger on spinous processes of lumbar spine to check for mobility.

- **Rotation** – Rock the pelvis with one hand, hook fingers of other hand into the spinous processes and pull/push to check for mobility.

8.3 <u>KNEE EXAMINATION</u>

<u>GENERAL</u>

The knee joint is a strong and stable **hinge joint**. The **cruciate ligaments** and **menisci** inside the joints and the **collateral ligaments** and **capsule** outside the joints along with **muscles** maintain knee stability when standing and moving.

Menisci are relatively unstable and susceptible to injury ("torn cartilage"). The knees are commonly affected by seronegative arthritis (psoriatic etc.), rheumatoid arthritis and osteoarthritis.

<u>INSPECTION</u>

- Observe for swelling, particularly the lateral and medial cavity (as in sepsis, OA/RA, gout or pseudo-gout).

- Observe quadriceps for wasting (usually the first sign in chronically painful knees – vastus lateralis, initially).

- The patient might lie on couch with the knee slightly flexed in extension. Limitation suggests flexion deformities e.g. hamstring tightness (or hip flexion problem); a locked knee with painful resistance suggest debris as in meniscal tear.

- Consider dermatomal pain and check hip (e.g. L3, L4 referred).

<u>PALPATION</u>

- Temperature – If hot, consider infection / inflammation.

- If swollen   - Does it feel bony? Consider OA; Does it feel boggy? Consider RA; Does it feel watery? Could be OA or RA.

- Mobilise patella – Is it fixed or mobile? If mobile, is it grinding? – Indicates early OA.

- Apply pressure under patella – Pain may indicate chondromalacia patellae.

- Patella tap test for fluid – Milk the infrapatellar bursa and suprapatellar bursa and tap patella. Movement and tapping sound can indicate effusion (normally little or no downward movement and tapping).

- Pressure on medial and lateral meniscus - If torn, it will be painful.

- Pressure on patellar tendon – Pain indicates tendonitis. To be sure, use isometric test to elicit pain response.

- Swelling in the popliteal fossa – Baker's cyst?

MOBILITY

- **Flexion** - Ask the patient to flex their knee and observe the extent of the angle – compare both knees. Use passive flexion if necessary.

- **Extension** - Fix the patient's thigh to the couch and test extension by pulling up the foot.

- Flex the patient's knee whilst watching their face for pain and feeling for crepitus. Is there any stiffness? Is it bouncy? – might be due to reflex muscle activity, i.e. a stroke may cause hyperreflexia; Is it bony? - probably OA.

STABILITY

- **Test lateral and medial collateral ligaments**. Must be tested with knee slightly bent so the leg joint is not bone-to-bone. Test with opposing pressures to feel for laxity or pain (Apparent lateral or medial movement with widening of joint line suggests weakness or tear).

- **Test anterior and posterior cruciate ligaments**. Flex the knee to 90°, ensure you stabilise the patient's foot on the couch and do not rotate the hip or tibia. Test by drawing the head of the tibia forward (and backward). Excessive movement suggests cruciate tear.

- **Test meniscus** (Mc Murray Test) – with the knee in 90-degree flexion, internally and externally rotate heel, all the time feeling the lateral and medial joint line. Apply pressure on the lateral aspect of the knee to create valgus stress and externally rotate and extend leg.

Note:
- To establish tendon injury, the tendon must be compromised by isometric pressure.

- To establish ligament damage requires movement of the joint.

8.4 <u>SHOULDER EXAMINATION</u>

<u>GENERAL</u>

The shoulder (a ball and socket joint) is functionally opposite to the knee. The knee is weight bearing and requires strong ligamentous support; it is stable and comparatively less mobile than the shoulder. The shoulder is non-weight bearing and requires minimum ligamentous support. It is more mobile than the knee and requires more muscular and tendinous support, and therefore sacrifices stability.

Note
When examining shoulders, always compare both sides: if limitations are the same on both side, then it is <u>possibly</u> normal; if they are different, something is wrong!

<u>INSPECTION</u>

- Look for inflammation (rubor, dolor, calor, functio-laesa), atrophy, discolouration and asymmetry.

<u>PALPATION</u>

Palpate the shoulder, head of humerus, bicipital groove, acromioclavicular joint (ACJ) and sternoclavicular (SCJ).

- Palpate for swellings and temperature, localise tenderness or pain by pressure around the joints.

- Pressure on tendon insertion - tenderness indicates tendonitis e.g. bicipital groove, head of humerus.

- Pressure on acromioclavicular joint (ACJ) – tenderness indicates arthritis.

<u>MOBILITY</u>

Active (Show the patient the movements and then get them to do it)

- Flexion-adduction (painful mid-arc suggests rotator cuff tendinitis and subacromial impingement).

- External rotation/internal rotation.

- Extension.

- External rotation and abduction (lift hand behind head).

- Internal rotation and extension (reach behind back).

- Scarf test – touch opposite shoulder (tenderness or pain at ACJ suggests arthritis).

Passive (You gently mobilise the patient's joints)

Sit the patient on the couch or chair and stand behind them holding their shoulder and wrist. As you mobilise, feel for **crepitus**, which may be due to degenerative changes in the acromioclavicular or glenohumeral joint.

- Flexion/abduction/adduction.

- Extension.

- External rotation, internal rotation.

- Hand behind head (External rotation/abduction.); Hand behind back (internal rotation/adduction).

Isometric tests of muscle and tendons

- Abduction against resistance – tests supraspinatus.

- Internal rotation against resistance – tests subscapularis.

- Lateral rotation against resistance – tests infraspinatus/teres minor.

- Adduction against resistance – tests axio-humoral.

- Elbow flexion against resistance – tests biceps (also inspect for a bulge in the muscle - rupture).

Notes

- Limitation of active movement **only**, suggests injury of muscles and tendons.

- Limitation of active **and** passive movement suggests joint pathology (bone, capsule or inflammation).

Common pathologies:

- Supraspinatus tendonitis. ⎤

- Subacromium bursitis. ⎬ 'Painful arc' sign

- Acromioclavicular arthritis. ⎦

- Adhesive capsulitis – Universal limitation and pain, particularly in external rotation / abduction.

- It is estimated that 70% of shoulder injuries are tendinitis.

When the above tests and findings prove negative, think away from the shoulder e.g. T1, T2, C5, etc. – spinal nerve damage; fibromyalgia; also, heart and gall bladder referred pain. Consider in conjunction with the patient's history.

8.5 HIP JOINT EXAMINATION

GENERAL

Except for gait inspection and Trendelenberg's test, examine with the patient lying on the couch. If the patient cannot lie down, methods can be adapted for examination with the patient seated.

INSPECTION

- Observe gait of 'stance and swing' (most problems appear during the weight bearing phase, i.e. stance). Hip dislocation, arthritis or abductor weakness, produces antalgic gait (short stance time on the painful leg) and abductor lurch (swaying the trunk far over the affected hip to minimise movement when walking because the pelvis tends to drop to the opposite side), aka. waddling gait.

- Trendelenberg's test – To test the right hip, the patient stands with their back to you and bends the left knee lifting it off floor. The hip should remain level or tilt to the right; this is a negative Trendelenberg's test. If the hip drops to the left it is a positive Trendelenberg's and there is severe hip disease with gluteal weakness.

- Look for inflammation - redness, swelling etc. and deformities, e.g. flexion, rotation, etc.

PALPATION

- Trochanteric bursa – Swelling and tenderness suggests bursitis. NB. Point tenderness over the trochanter is an essential finding but tenderness above (superior) suggests gluteus medius tendinitis.

- Along inguinal ligament – Bulges may be hernia or aneurism; Enlarged lymph nodes suggest infection of pelvis or lower limbs; Tenderness may be hip synovitis, iliopsoas bursitis or psoas abscess.

- Ischiogluteal bursa – If swollen and tender, suggests bursitis.

MOBILITY

Passive

- **Flexion** – Flex the hip, it should normally achieve 120°. Watch for drag of pelvis upwards (In OA the joint commonly locks and compensates with a pelvic tilt).

- **Abduction** – Stabilise the pelvis and abduct the leg (watch the pelvis does not move outward – not true abduction). Figure 4 is a useful test for abduction and external rotation. NB. Abduction and external rotation are lost early on in arthritis.

- **Adduction** – Stabilise the pelvis and cross one leg over the other.

- **External and internal rotation** – Lift the patient's knee at right angle, hold the knee and rotate the leg medially (ext.rot.); lift the knee at right angle and rotate laterally (int.rot.). Should achieve 45° rotation (Pain and limited movement are an early and reliable sign of hip disease).

- **Extension** – With patient prone, secure their sacrum and lift the leg.

Active

Observe and note any pain and limitation of movement in:

- Flexion / extension.

- Adduction / abduction.

- External rotation / internal rotation.

Note: Hip pathology may be felt at the knee (This is referred pain because it has the same nerve root, L2 and L3). In females, cyclic hip pain might indicate endometriosis.

8.6 ELBOW EXAMINATION

GENERAL

The elbow provides a link between the powerful movements of the shoulder and the fine motor control of the hand. It is comprised of three bones, the **humerus radius** and **ulna**. The humerus expands into **condyles**

Three primary nerves cross the elbow (radial, medial and ulnar). Their relatively superficial course in the elbow and distal portion of the forearm predispose them to acute, traumatic injury.

Several **bursae** are found in the elbow region. The **subcutaneous olecranon bursa** is commonly injured in sports but the **sub-tendinous olecranon bursa** may become inflamed secondary to repetitive stress.

INSPECTION

- Look for scars, contusions, swelling – Tendon rupture (in antecubital fossa)? Olecranon process – bursitis? Grossly deformed – dislocation or fracture (Sudden swelling and pain without trauma may indicate gout or RA)?

- Inspect forearm angle (Palms forward and at side). Normally show an outward angle of 5° - 8°. A negative angle suggests malunion or supracondylar fracture.

PALPATION

- Palpate the ligaments for tenderness.

- Palpate the olecranon bursa (Not palpable unless inflamed).

- Ulnar nerve palpation or light tapping in the ulnar groove may induce paraesthesia's in the forearm or ulnar two fingers – Suggests entrapment.

- Palpate the lateral epicondyle whilst the patient flexes their wrist – Point tenderness and crepitus indicates lateral epicondylitis (Tennis elbow).

- Palpate the lateral epicondyle with resisted wrist extension – Pain indicates epicondylitis.

- Palpate the medial epicondyle while the patient extends their wrist – Point tenderness and crepitus indicates medial epicondylitis (golfer's elbow or medial tennis elbow).

- Palpate the lateral epicondyle with resisted wrist flexion – Pain indicates medial epicondylitis.

NB. Correlate with other findings as the condyle and ulnar nerve are normally sensitive).

MOBILITY

- Normal flexion 0-130°; Normal pronation/supination 80° each way; normal extension 0°. but may be a slight angle, especially in female athletes.
  (Active testing may suffice if not, perform passive tests).

- Stiffness indicates any of the abnormalities mentioned above.

STABILITY

- Test for valgus and varus stress - Pain or laxity may indicate sports injuries.

9. NEUROLOGICAL EXAMINATION
(See Bates: Chapter 18)

GENERAL

A complete neurological examination requires in-depth knowledge of the nervous system. For Herbalists, a more general knowledge is required so that one understands the basic findings to know when to refer the patient to their GP or specialist, or to be able to recognise improvement or otherwise, as a result of one's treatments in a known condition. To this end, one should have a sound knowledge and understanding of the anatomy and physiology of the nervous system (Refer to any Tortura *et al*).

Neurologically, the patient may present with one or more of several symptoms and signs:

SYMPTOMS	SIGNS
Pain (most common)	Pain
Weakness (common)	Abnormal gait
Paraesthesia (important)	Flaccidity/spasticity
Anaesthesia	Atrophy
Immobility	Immobility
Tremor	Tremor

Side note: Pain might well be neural in origin but also think about other causes, e.g. in the legs, pain might result from intermittent claudication or deep vein thrombosis. Knowing, the signs, symptoms and history will help differential diagnosis.

Be aware that:
Claudication – Stops the patient walking. Examine pulse and colour. Look around eyes for xanthelasma or corneal arcus (indicates atherosclerosis).

Venous thrombosis – Results from prolonged immobility, post-surgery, the pill or trauma.

9.1 <u>MOTOR FUNCTION IN LIMBS</u>

Generally testing for **bulk, tone, strength**:

- **Bulk** – Look for atrophy and flaccidity

- **Tone** – Mobilise to look for deficit of tone or spasticity or clonus.

- **Strength** – Test for muscle power i.e. resist with pressure against movement and compare sides.

But **reflex** and **sensation/pain** are also part of the picture:

- **Reflex** – If weakness is found, use a reflex hammer to establish if the problem is Upper Motor Neurone (UMN) or Lower Motor Neurone (LMN).

- **Sensation** – If necessary, and with great care, try to elicit pain or paraesthesia to establish if the problem is nerve compression.

Note. Always compare sides.

<u>GENERAL OBSERVATION</u>

1. As the patient enters, look for abnormalities of gait or posture, e.g.

- **Spastic hemiparesis** – An arm and hand held immobile and flexed. The leg on same side extended with plantar flexion. Dragging of the same foot or circling outwards - Stroke.

- **Stepping gait** – Drags feet or lifts high and slaps down (like walking upstairs) - Lower Motor Neurone disease.

- **Parkinsonian gait** – Stooped head, hips and knees flexed with short shuffling steps. Slow to start and slow to stop - Disease of the basal ganglia i.e. Parkinson's.

- **Sensory ataxia** – Unsteady walking, needs to watch the ground, obvious heel/toe walking - Polyneuropathy or disease of the posterior column.

- **Cerebellar ataxia** – Staggering gait, wide base, exaggerated turns - Cerebellar stroke or tumour.

2. Look for abnormalities of higher brain functions, e.g.

- Lowered consciousness; disorientation of time, place, person; memory deficits – Consider organic lesions.

- Severe disturbance of mood or perception of reality – Consider psychiatric disorder.

INSPECTION

- **Bulk** – Look for atrophy (loss of muscle bulk) – Disuse? LMN disease e.g. Polio or Compression? UMN disease, e.g. MND?

- **Tone** – Mobilise the limb to look for deficit of tone or spasticity (increased resistance that varies)

  o **Increased** – Pyramidal lesion, e.g. established stroke ('clasp knife' i.e. catches then relaxes during rapid passive mobility like a spring-loaded clasp [pen] knife); Extrapyramidal, e.g. Parkinson's ('Lead pipe' or 'cogwheel' rigidity throughout passive mobility).

  o **Decreased** - Very recent stroke? LMN damage? Cerebellar damage?

  o **Paratonia** (Sudden changes - i.e. sudden loss and sudden increase) – Dementia?

MUSCLE STRENGTH TESTS

After testing for bulk and tone then test for muscle strength by resisting patient's movements with opposing pressure and compare both sides - testing for abnormal **paresis** (weakness).

- When carrying out the examination make clear to the patient what you require of them e.g. "Bend your elbow like this... Don't allow me to straighten it..." and signal readiness to them e.g. a finger tap or word.

- Use your body weight in a steady manner to apply pressure, don't tug.

- In all cases the patient resists your movement.

- Inform the patient to relax when you finish do not suddenly let go.

- Sometimes performed with the patient on the couch but sitting on a chair is usually sufficient.

Technique tip.

When testing, you can vary your strength and method in relation to the patient's strength, e.g. when testing biceps:

Practitioner's hand position:

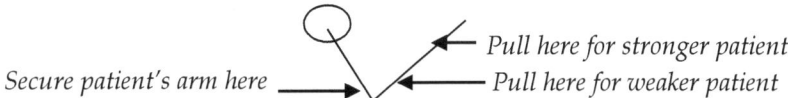

Secure patient's arm here ——→   ←— Pull here for stronger patient
←————— Pull here for weaker patient

State of patient's arm flexion:

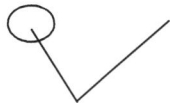

a) Optimum position of strength in arm - weaker patient at an advantage.

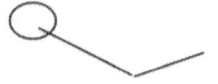 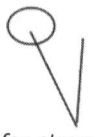

b) Either of these flexion states confer reduced capacity for strength – use for stronger patient, gives weaker practitioner an advantage.

NB Neurology is a very specialist skill. For general purposes, the following tests are indicators of muscular weaknesses related to the motor nerves given in brackets.

UPPER LIMB TESTS

- **Shoulder abduction** (deltoids assisted by supraspinatus – C5,6) Press down on the patient's outstretched arms.

- **Shoulder adduction** (pectoralis major – C6,7,8, T1; latissimus dorsi – C6,7,8) Place a steadying hand on the patient's shoulder and resist adduction by pulling against their elbow with your other hand.

- **Elbow flexion** (biceps, brachioradialis, brachialis – C5,6) Place a steadying hand on the elbow of the patient's flexed arm and with your other hand at the patient's wrist pull it toward you.

- **Elbow extension** (triceps – C6,7,8) Place a steadying hand on the elbow of the patient's flexed arm and with your other hand at the patient's wrist push it toward the patient.

LOWER LIMB TESTS

- **Hip flexion** (iliopsoas – L2,.3,4) Place a hand on the patient's thigh and ask them to push up.

- **Hip extension** (gluteus maximus– L5, S1,2) Place a hand underneath their bent knee and ask the patient to push down.

- **Hip abduction** (gluteus medius/minimus, tensor fasciae latae – L4,5, S1) Place hands outside both the patient's knees and ask them to push outwards.

- **Hip adduction** (adductors – L2,3,4) Place the hands inside the patient's knees and ask them to push inwards.

- **Knee extension** (quadriceps – L2,3,4) Place a steadying hand on the patient's flexed knee and the resisting hand on the ankle, then get them get to extend the leg.

- **Knee flexion** (biceps femoris – L4,5 S1,2) With a steadying hand on their flexed knee and resisting hand behind their ankle, get the patient to increase flexion.

- **Foot Dorsiflexion** (L4,5) With their legs full extended, ask the patient to pull their feet up against your hands.

- **Plantar flexion** (S1) With their legs full extended, ask the patient to push against your hands.

ADDITIONAL TESTS TO ESTABLISH UMN OR LMN LESION

Sensation – If weakness is found, you might try to elicit pain or paraesthesia to establish compression pathology and therefore, LMN damage.

1. Femoral Nerve Test
The femoral nerve arises from L1, L2 and L3, it comes under the inguinal ligament and innervates the quadriceps – stretch it by extending hip and ask if there is any pain (In the back or leg) or tap on it.

2. Sciatic Nerve Test
The sciatic nerve arises from L4, L5, S1, S2 and S3, and innervates everything except the quadriceps. Whilst observing the patient, raise the straightened leg slowly and look for pain (SLR – straight leg raise). To ensure it is not facet joint or muscle stretch pain, lower the leg just below the point of pain and dorsiflex the foot. If pain occurs, then this suggests nerve root compression.

Note: The less the angle of raising, the more severe the root compression.

Reflex testing

After testing bulk, tone, strength and sensation (nerve stretch), if weakness is found, use a reflex hammer to establish if UMN or LMN lesion. A useful way to remember the basic innervation of the limbs is:

S1, 2 - Ankle
L3, 4 - Knee
C5, 6 - Biceps
C7, 8 - Triceps

Note. Distinctions between UMN and LMN lesions can often be assisted by the following signs, which are the result of either loss of UMN innervation/control or LMN innervation/control:

Sign	UMN lesion	LMN lesion	Reason
Flaccid paralysis	√ Early		Lack of UMN innervation
Spastic paralysis	√		Lack of descending control
Hypertonia	√		Lack of descending control
Hyperreflexia	√		Lack of descending control of reflex arc
Clonus	√		Lack of descending control of reflex arc
Flaccid hypotonia		√	Lack of LMN innervation
Atrophy	√	√	Lack of innervation and activity
Early atrophy		√	Lack of LMN innervation and nutrition / metabolic integrity
Fasciculation	Widespread in MND	√	Due to contraction of single motor units
Hyporeflexia, Areflexia	√ Early	√	Loss of reflex arc

Examples of LMN lesions: disc compression, polio, peripheral neuropathy.

Examples of UMN lesions: stroke, MS, MND, tumour, cord compression.

- Acute lesions of the pyramidal tract (e.g. stroke) causes flaccid paralysis and areflexia initially. However, increased tone follows within several days due to loss of descending control of spinal reflex activity resulting in spastic paralysis and hyperreflexia.

- Weakness of muscles might be due to 1) lack of use. 2) dominant use of one side. 3) lower motor neurone damage (e.g. root compression). 4) upper motor neurone damage (e.g. stroke, MS).

- With MS or stroke (UMN lesions), muscles may be tight, whereas in LMN damage muscles may be just weak.

- Flaccidity and atrophy may be due to lack of innervation resulting from UMN or LMN lesions. However, LMN cell bodies supply nutritional protein and therefore, atrophy is more obvious and rapid in LMN lesions.

EXAMPLES OF MOTOR NEURONE DISORDERS

Multiple Sclerosis

Multiple demyelination in brain and spinal cord. Predilection for:

- o Optic nerves - optic neuropathy, blurred vision, mild ocular pain, optic neuritis.

- o Brain stem and cerebellar connections - diplopia, vertigo facial numbness, dysphagia.

- o Chord lesions (particularly cervical chord) - spastic paraparesis, difficulty walking, sensory disturbances, urinary symptoms.

- o Paraventricular regions.

- Common onset, age 20 – 35 (More common in women).

- Some familial incidence.

- Wasting unusual due to sparing of anterior horn.

Motor Neurone disease

Progressive degeneration of motor neurones in spinal cord and somatic motor nuclei of cranial nerves and within cortex:

- Unknown cause, 6:100 000, slight male predominance, occurs in middle life.

- There are three patterns which may merge later in disease progression:

    1. Progressive muscular atrophy (Fasciculation common).

    2. Amyotrophic lateral sclerosis (Spastic paresis with atrophy).

    3. Progressive bulbar palsy – dysarthria, dysphagia, nasal regurgitation of fluids, and choking.

Myasthenia gravis

Immune destruction of acetylcholine receptors:

- Weakness of proximal limbs, ocular and bulbar muscles – mastication speech, facial expression, respiration.

- Muscle wasting sometimes seen late on in disease.

- Occurrence: 4:100000; 2 x more common in women: Any age - peak incidence, 30.

Muscular dystrophy

Progressively genetically determined disorder of skeletal and sometimes cardiac muscle:

- 1:3000 male infants.

- Causes death by age 20

- Marked by weakness and wasting of skeletal muscle.

- Pseudo-hypertrophy of calves and later on shoulders and upper limbs.

9.2 **SENSORY ASSESSMENT**

GENERAL

Conventionally, sensory examination begins distally and moves proximally up the limb. Sensory deficit should fit into four main categories:

1. **Global sensory loss** – Entire limb, e.g. stroke.

2. **Peripheral neuropathy** – 'Glove and stocking' distribution, e.g. diabetes, alcoholism.

3. **Dermatomal sensory loss** - Single dermatomes, e.g. nerve root compression; Two or more in a peripheral nerve distribution, e.g. ulnar nerve as in ulnar nerve entrapment.

4. **Dissociated sensory loss** – Loss of certain sensory modalities but preservation of others such as loss of pain and temperature sensation but intact light touch and proprioception, e.g. syringomyelia (expansion of the spinal cord cavity affects the spinothalamic tract but the dorsal column is not affected).

- Sensory testing is complex and requires a good knowledge of neural pathways and dermatomes (Learn the basic **dermatomes**, **peripheral nerves** and the **spinothalamic tract** and **dorsal column**). However, there are basic patterns and tests that help us identify sensory deficits and consequently enable us to refer or assess levels of improvement.

- When testing, first inform the patient about what you are going to do and what you expect from them, then ask the patient to keep their eyes closed throughout.

- When testing sensations, compare both sides.

- When an area of sensory deficit or hypersensitivity is located try to map out its boundary. Thus, you can infer the origin of the lesion and possibly its cause.

- When abnormal findings are detected you may need to correlate them with any motor or reflex abnormality.

TESTING VIBRATION, PROPRIOCEPTION AND LIGHT TOUCH

Deficit suggests **dorsal column** sensory loss although damage to any sensory component from the skin to the cortex will lead to deficit.

Light touch

- Ask the patient to close their eyes.

- Dab the sternum with a piece of cotton wool, ask patient if they can feel it and that it feels soft as they would expect cotton wool to feel.

- Dab the fingers and lateral and medial aspect of the arms and compare stimulus across the dermatomes. Ask patient to say "yes" if it feels the same.

- If an area of deficit is identified dab again to confirm your findings and then proceed to map out the area.

Vibration (Using a suitable tuning fork – 128Hz)

Deficit is an early sign of neuropathy, i.e. a nerve is unable to conduct discrete impulses.

- Hold an activated fork over the patient's sternum to identify vibration – tell the patient to identify the 'buzzing' not the pressure.

- Place an activated tuning fork firmly over the distal interphalangeal joint of the patient's thumb (C6) and big toe (L5) of both sides. Ask 'What do you feel?".

- If uncertain whether the patient identifies pressure or vibration, ask the patient to tell you when the vibration stops and then touch the tuning fork to dampen vibration.

- If sensory findings are intact at the periphery, they are usually intact proximally.

- If sensory impairment is found distally, proceed proximally, e.g. wrist (T1, C6-8), elbow (T1, C6); medial malleolus (L4), patella (L3); ASIS (L1), spinous processes and clavicles (C3/4).

Deficits might indicate: peripheral neuropathy, e.g. alcoholism, diabetes, dorsal column disease e.g. tertiary syphilis or B12 deficiency.

Proprioception (Joint position sense - JPS) – The ability to sense (via stretch receptors) the position of the joint in space.

Like vibration sense, if intact at the periphery it is usually intact proximally.

- Grasp the proximal phalanx of the patient's thumb between your thumb and finger of one hand and with the other hand grasp the distal phalanx. Show the patient the intended "up or down" movement.

- With the patient's eyes closed, wiggle the distal phalanx a few times and stop in either position asking the patient to indicate the position they think it is in.

- If they identify correctly move to the other hand. If they identify incorrectly check again to confirm and then move to the other digits and next proximal joints.

- Next grasp the proximal phalanx of patient's big toe between your thumb finger of one hand and with the other grasp the distal phalanx. Show the patient the intended "up or down" movement.

- With the patient's eyes closed, wiggle the distal phalanx a few times (avoiding contact with other toes) and stop in either position asking the patient to indicate the position they think it is in. Move proximally if incorrect.

- Also, consider using Romberg's test.

TESTING PAIN, TEMPERATURE AND CRUDE TOUCH

Deficit suggests **spinothalamic tract** sensory loss.

Test proximal and distal areas of the limbs as in light touch but ensure you cover:

- Both shoulders (C5); lateral/medial forearms (C6, T1); thumbs and little fingers (C6-C8).

- Front of thighs (L2); medial/lateral calves (L4, L5); little toe (S1); medial buttocks (S3).

Pain

- Use something that gives a sharp sensation as a surrogate for pain.

- Response may be subjective, so test on the patient's sternum as a baseline for sharpness (Warn the patient you are using something sharp and gently tap on the skin and get them to confirm it feels sharp).

- Apply the lightest pressure needed to the areas and <u>do not draw blood</u>.

- Move on to the fingers and arms as in light touch but ask them to confirm "sharp" or "dull" if this is the case.

- Compare sides, "Does this feel the same as this?"

- Safely discard the tool after use.

Temperature (Not routinely tested)

- Ask the patient to close their eyes.

- Touch the patient with a cold tuning fork and get them to identify the quality of the sensation (A crude test used clinically).

- For greater discrimination use a warm and a cool instrument touch the area and ask "is it hot or cold".

Two-point discrimination

Use an opened paper clip and apply pressure to an area and ask if one or two points were applied.

Minimal distances for normal ability to discriminate two points:

Upper arm and thigh -- 75mm
Back -- 40-70mm
Fingertips -- 2-8mm
Toes -- 3-8mm
Palm -- 8-12mm
Chest and forearm -- 40mm
Tongue -- 1mm

In disease states, such as peripheral neuropathy, the distance at which two points can normally perceived is increased, in some cases by several centimetres.

CORTICAL (DISCRIMINATIVE) SENSORY TESTS

If peripheral sensory functions are intact but individuals present with sensory abnormalities, the following tests may be useful in identifying cortical dysfunction:

- **Point localisation** – Ask the patient (With their eyes closed) to localise tactile stimuli.

- **Stereognosis** – Ask the patient (With their eyes closed) to identify objects placed in their hand e.g. a coin etc.

- **Graphaesthesia** – Use a blunt instrument to trace digits on the palm of the patient's hand and ask them to identify it.

- **Two-point discrimination** - Use an opened paper clip and apply pressure to an area and ask if one or two points were applied.

9.3 <u>COORDINATION (some sensory)</u>

- **Patient's arms out in front, eyes closed for 20 – 30 seconds** (standing or seated)

  - Pronation of arm with downward drift – Pyramidal weakness?

  - Sideward or upward drift – Loss of position sense? cerebellar dysfunction?

  - Tremors – Parkinson's disease (course resting tremor– reduces on movement)? Thyrotoxicosis (fine tremor)?

- **Tap the patient's arms downward** (Arms in front, eyes closed, instruct the patient to return arms to position)

  - Easily displaced and remains so - Arm weakness?

  - Correction poor - Sensory weakness?

  - Overshoots and bounces - Cerebellar dysfunction.

- **Romberg's test** – (Standing, feet together, arms at the side, eyes open then closed)

  - Ataxia with eyes closed – Suggests dorsal column sensory loss.

  - Ataxia with eyes open or closed (Positive Romberg's) – Cerebellar ataxia

- **Finger to nose test**

  - Intention tremors – Suggests cerebellar dysfunction.

  - Past pointing – Suggests cerebellar dysfunction.

- **Alternating hand movements**

  - Dysdiadokinesia – Suggests cerebellar dysfunction.

- **Fast finger movement with arms out** (Piano fingers)

  - Clumsy – Mild pyramidal weakness?

- **Heel to shin test**

  - Heel overshoots knee and oscillates on shin – Cerebellar dysfunction.

  - Heel lifted too high, (Patient needs to look); worse with eyes closed – Sensory loss.

9.4 <u>DEEP TENDON REFLEX</u>

Reflexes vary from person to person and some are more difficult to elicit than others. Having been shown how to perform this technique, you will only become proficient with practice.

Indications of abnormal reflexes:

• Reduced or pendular - Cerebellar dysfunction.

• Increased - UMN lesion.

• Reduced or absent - LMN lesion

Notes

• If reflexes are hyperactive, test for clonus. (Normal people control antagonism of stretch reflex with UMN, clonus occurs in UMN dysfunction).

• If reflexes are symmetrically diminished or absent, use reinforcement techniques (Jendrassic manoeuvre).

• General muscle innervation:

> *Biceps C5, C6*
> *Triceps C6, C7*
> *Supinator C5, C6*
> *Knee L2, L3, L4*
> *Ankle S1*
> *Abdominal T8, T9, T10*
> *Plantar (Babinski sign) L5, S1*

9.5 <u>CRANIAL NERVE EXAMINATION</u>

The following is a basic guide. You should study the pathologies and techniques in relevant texts.

CN I Olfactory

- Ask the patient to seal off one nostril and breathe in to ensure clear nasal passage in the other. Then, with their eyes closed ask them to inhale a substance with a well-known smell (coffee or lemon) and ask them what they can smell (both sides).

- Loss of smell (anosmia) may be due to head trauma, infection, smoking, blockage, cocaine. Nasal hallucinations may be due to chronic sinusitis, infection or temporal lobe tumour - the patient might complain of noticing a burning smell.

CN II Optic

- **Visual acuity** – Using a Snellen chart, the patient should be able to read the sixth line at six metres (20 feet) People who wear glasses should have them on.

  When using this chart, the lowest line of letters the subject can read is noted. The line read is recorded as a fraction, e.g. 6/60, 6/5, 6/6 this is known as Snellen acuity.

  The top number, usually 6, means the distance at which the test was carried out i.e. 6 metres. The bottom number is the smallest size of letters the subject could read.

  The largest letter on the Snellen chart is usually 60. A person only able to read this line at six metres has poor vision. A person with normal vision could read it at 60 metres (200 feet).

  The smallest letters are usually 5. A person able to read this line at 6 metres has better than normal vision. A person with normal visual acuity could only read it at 5 metres (16 feet).

NORMAL VISION is 6/6, 6 is usually the next to the bottom line (or on some charts two lines up from the bottom) (In the USA, normal vision is called 20/20).

- **Mapping visual fields** – Start by mapping the blind spot. Confront the patient (from approximately 1 meter/yard). With each covering the directly opposing eyes on one side, map the blind spot by moving a coloured pin head from the lateral to the medial aspect of the horizontal field of vision and ask the patient to indicate when the pinhead disappears and reappears (An enlarged area, compared to yours which should be normal, is a feature of papilloedema). Then test the other eye.

  Next (using the same position), starting from outside the field of vision, bring your moving finger throughout the four quadrants to locate any loss of vision over the fields. Then test the other eye.

- **Pupillary reflex** (also tests CNIII) – Tests direct and indirect reflex to locate II or III nerve damage.

  Use a pen torch brought from the outside the field of vision to shine on the pupil and look for the reaction to the additional light, which should normally be bilateral constriction (Test both sides).

  Some examples of abnormalities: Tonic pupil, i.e. large/unilateral - reaction reduced/absent; Oculomotor nerve paralysis - dilated pupil fixed to light and near effort, possible ptosis and lateral deviation; Horner's syndrome - constricted pupil although reacts briskly to light and near effort; Argyll-Robertson - both pupils constricted and unreactive to light, but do react to near effort.

- **Ophthalmoscopy** – To detect optic atrophy (death of optic nerve fibres) and papilloedema.

Notes.

Most problems are refractory, not optic nerve. However, total loss of field in one eye may be due to pathology of cornea, lens, vitreous body, retina or optic nerve in front of optic chiasm. Bitemporal hemianopsia may be due to pituitary tumour. Homonymous hemianopsia may be due to damage to the optic tract.

CN III Oculomotor, IV Trochlear, VI Abducens

- Ocular muscles - Ensure the patient keeps their head still and ask them to follow your finger with their eyes (you are trying to detect minimal weakness) as you move it in all directions. Hold the finger still at the ends of directions to see if there is any weakness. Look for nystagmus and strabismus and ask if they see double.

- Accommodation and convergence (CNIII) – Ask the patient to look out of the window and place a pen in front at about 1 metre, then say 'look at the pen' as you bring it right up to the nose. Observe pupillary constriction and convergence (medial rectus).

CN V Trigeminal

- Motor function – Palpate the temporalis and ask the patient to clench their teeth; palpate the masseters and ask the patient to clench their teeth; secure the patients jaw and ask them to open against resistance; ask the patient to close their jaw against resistance; ask the patient to push their jaw sideways against resistance (tests pterygoids).

- Sensory function – With a soft brush, stroke the ophthalmic, maxillary and mandibular regions and compare both sides. Ask the patient, 'Do you feel that?' 'Do they feel the same on both sides?' Also, test temperature (with a cold object) and, if required, use something that gives a sharp sensation as a surrogate for pain. **NB. Avoid testing this nerve if the patient suffers from trigeminal neuralgia**

- Corneal reflex (sensory CNV, motor CNVII) - Important fibres in the ophthalmic division are the corneal fibres (reflex is lost in certain tumours). Test by brushing the cornea with a wisp of cotton wool. Ask the patient to look up and away from you as you approach out of the patient's line of vision: The patient should blink on gentle touch.

CN VII Facial
- Facial symmetry – Ask the patient to make facial expressions, e.g. smile, frown, etc. Distortion, i.e. a lack of expression on one side may indicate Bell's Palsy (in LMN VII lesion, the whole side is affected) or stroke (in UMN VII lesion, the upper facial muscles spared due to bilateral innervation).

- Taste – There are various tests, but a convenient method is to brush a vitamin C tablet on tongue to see if the patient can taste it.

CN VIII Vestibulocochlear
- Hearing loss – You should know that bone conducts sound better than air. However, the mechanisms of the ear are much more sensitive to sound transmitted through the air. Also, remember the patient will be telling you which ear is problematic; you must establish whether it is **conductive** or **sensorineural** deafness.

- **Rinne's test** (comparing air and bone conduction) - Place the vibrating tuning fork on the mastoid bone and ask the patient if they can hear it. When the patient can no longer hear it, place the U of the fork close to the ear. Normally sound is heard longer through air than through bone. In conductive loss, sound is heard through bone as long or longer than through air, therefore, there would be no sound heard at the canal. In sensorineural hearing loss, sound, if heard at all, is heard longer through air than bone just as in normal hearing. NB there are variations of this test.

- **Weber's test** (for lateralisation) – Place the base of the vibrating fork on top of the patient's head in the centre. Ask where they hear it, normally it is heard on both sides but in unilateral sensorineural deafness, sound is heard best in the good ear. In conductive deafness sound is heard best in the bad ear because all extraneous noise is blocked out.

CN IX Glossopharyngeal, CN X Vagus
Ask the patient to say 'Ah' and watch for symmetrical movement of the palate (The palate will move away from the side of a lesion). Check the patient can swallow and cough.

CN XI Spinal accessory
Test the power of the sternomastoid and trapezius by resisting the patient's shoulder shrug (trapezius) and resisting turning of the head (sternomastoid)

CN XII Hypoglosseal
Ask patient to protrude their tongue. It should be symmetrical (The tongue will deviate to the side of the lesion). Wasting and fasciculation indicates a LMN lesion.

10. <u>KIDNEY AND URINARY TRACT</u>

The primary function of the kidneys is to filter metabolic waste, excess Na^+ and H_2O and to help eliminate them from the body. They also play an important role in regulation of blood pressure and RBC production.

Each kidney has a ureter, which drains urine from the kidney into the bladder. From the bladder, the urine passes through the urethra in the penis in males and the vulva in females.

<u>SYMPTOMS OF URINARY TRACT DISORDERS.</u>

Fever

Common symptoms of disorders are fever and malaise, consider that:

- Bladder infections (cystitis) generally do not cause fever.

- Bacterial infection of kidneys (pyelonephritis) causes high fever.

- Kidney cancer occasionally causes fever.

Frequency (Frequent urination without an increase in total daily amount i.e. more than normal frequency of 4-6 times per day)

- Bladder infection? Foreign body irritating bladder e.g. stone or tumour?

- Nocturia (Frequency at night) Kidney disease? CHF? Liver failure? Diabetes? Drinking excess fluid late in the evening?

- Enlarged prostate.

Dysuria (Painful urination)

- Bladder irritation/infection?

Urgency (Compelling need to urinate. Amount usually small - control is lost if unable to urinate).

- Bladder irritation/infection.

Enuresis (bedwetting – normal up to age 3)

- Infection or narrowing of urethra.

- Neurogenic bladder (inadequate control of nerves of bladder: genetic or psychological).

Difficulty Starting accompanied by need to strain, weak stream, difficulty stopping (dribble).

- Enlarged prostate or less commonly urethral stricture.

- Abnormally narrow urethra in women and boys.

Incontinence (Unintentional passing of urine)

- Cystocele (herniation of bladder into vagina from weakening of pelvic muscles during childbirth or changes resulting from oestrogen reduction at menopause).

- Obstruction outflow (causes excess pressure in bladder).

Polyuria (Passage of large volumes of urine with an increase in urinary frequency)

- Diabetes.

- Diabetes insipidus and nephrogenic diabetes insipidus.

Pain caused by kidney disease

- Usually in the flank or small of back

Pain caused by stone entering ureter

- Severe cramping pain in the lower back entering the groin.

Pain caused by bladder infection

- Usually suprapubic and at the outer end of the urethra during urination. (Suprapubic pain may also be due to also outflow obstruction)

DIAGNOSTIC PROCEDURES

During palpation, the kidneys cannot normally be felt, but a swollen kidney, swollen bladder or tumour might be detectable. GPs and some Herbalists will perform a rectal examination of the prostate. A vaginal examination might provide information about the bladder and urethra.

Additional tests might include dipstick and microscopic urine analysis, blood tests that reflect kidney function, imaging procedures and cell sampling. However, Herbalists are limited to dipstick analysis.

Although some obvious diseases are mentioned here, you should be aware that virtually every medical condition that could present in humans might reflect in abnormal values of various urinary substances.

DIPSTICK TESTING

GLUCOSE
Abnormal values might indicate:
Diabetes mellitus? Excessive consumption of carbohydrates? Occasionally stress (adrenaline stimulates gluconeogenesis)? Renal glycosuria? Renal glycosuria during pregnancy?

BILIRUBIN
Haemoglobin breakdown results in bilirubin production. The liver normally conjugates it and therefore prevents it being absorbed in the gut. If prevented from entering the duodenum conjugated bilirubin, being water-soluble, returns to the blood and is excreted in urine.

Abnormal values might indicate:
Obstruction of bile duct/biliary tree.

KETONES
Produced by the body when fat is being used for energy e.g. during starvation. As they are acidic they may be harmful in excess.

Abnormal values might indicate:
Diabetic ketoacidosis? Insulin overdose? Starvation? Nausea and vomiting? Strict dieting? Severe stress? Severe fever due to infection?

NB. If glucose and ketones are present immediate action is required, i.e. REFER.

SPECIFIC GRAVITY
Measures the amount of substances dissolved in the urine. It also indicates how well the kidneys can adjust the amount of water in urine. The higher the specific gravity, the more solid material is dissolved in the urine. Intake of high volumes of water produces greater-than-normal amounts of dilute urine. Intake of low volumes of water produces only small amounts of concentrated urine.

Abnormal values:

- **Reduced** (Dilute) - Diabetes insipidus? Renal diseases (loss of ability to reabsorb water)? Excess fluid intake?

- **Raised** – (Concentrated) Dehydration? Excessive sweating? Diarrhoea? Liver disease?

NB. A random sample between 1.002 and 1.030 should be considered normal in the absence of kidney disease. Measurements below 1.010 indicate hydration, measurements above this figure indicate relative dehydration.

pH
Blood filtrate is usually acidified by kidneys from 7.4 to 6, but pH varies considerably with diet.

- *Persistent alkaline >7* – Vegetarian? UTI? Urinary tract obstruction? Pyloric stenosis/vomiting? Respiratory alkalosis? Alkalising drugs?

- *Persistent acid <7* - High protein diet? Gout? Fever? Starvation and dehydration? Uncontrolled diabetes? Predisposition to uric acid calculi (kidney stones)? Respiratory acidosis?

Notes.
Most bacteria responsible for UTIs tend to make urine more alkaline (splits urea to ammonia etc.).

Decreased ventilation occurs during sleep therefore, the first specimen is usually highly acidic.

BLOOD
Abnormal values might indicate:
Acute inflammation of urinary organs due to kidney and bladder calculi? Damage to kidney and bladder? Tumours? Kidney disease? Haemolytic disease? Menstrual blood?

Consider that:
- Blood seen at start of voiding suggests bleeding from the urethra.

- Blood throughout voiding suggests blood from the bladder or higher up.

- Blood at the end of voiding suggests bleeding from the prostate or bladder base.

- Haematuria + frequency + urgency suggests infection.

- Haematuria + urinary tract pain suggests stones, infection, trauma.

- Haematuria + reduced renal function suggests nephritis.

- Painless haematuria raises suspicion of malignancy.

PROTEIN
Abnormal values might indicate:
- **Benign proteinurea**: Postural? Excess exercise? High or low temperature? Pregnancy?

- **Pathological proteinurea**: Colic? Cirrhosis? Pyelonephritis? Glomerulonephritis?

UROBILINOGEN
In the intestines, bacteria convert bilirubin to urobilinogen. This is then excreted and some is reabsorbed and passes to the liver and urine.

Abnormal values indicate:
Overburdening of liver? Haemolytic disease? Restricted liver function? Hepatic infection? Cirrhosis?

NITRITE
Gram -ve bacteria in urine reduces dietary nitrate to nitrite, forming the basis of this test.

Abnormal values might indicate:
Urinary tract infection? Bacterial infection, e.g. *E. coli*, salmonella?

If the patient is generally healthy, the problem may be cystitis or other infections. If the patient is generally unwell for a while, it might indicate tumour with infection.

LEUKOCYTES
Abnormal values might indicate:
Kidney infection? Cystitis? Urethritis? Vaginal secretions?

CHARACTER OF URINE

Colour

Many factors affect urine colour, including fluid balance, diet, medications, and disease. Pale or colourless urine indicates it is dilute, on the other hand deep-yellow urine indicates it is concentrated. Bright yellow urine indicates the patient is taking Vitamin B supplements. Reddish-brown urine indicates certain medications, blackberries, beetroot, or blood in the urine.

Clarity - Also called opacity or turbidity i.e. the cloudiness of urine.

Urine is normally clear. Bacteria, blood, sperm, crystals, or mucus can make urine appear cloudy.

Odour

Some diseases can cause a change in the normal odour of urine. For example, an infection with *E. coli* bacteria can cause a foul odour, while diabetes or starvation can cause a sweet, fruity odour.

APPENDIX 1.   <u>IDENTIFICATION OF PULSES</u>

What is a pulse?

1. When the heart contracts a surge of blood flows through the arteries

2. The surge distends the arteries, which contain elastic tissue

3. The stretch and subsequent recoil of the arteries travels in a wave. This is the **pulse**

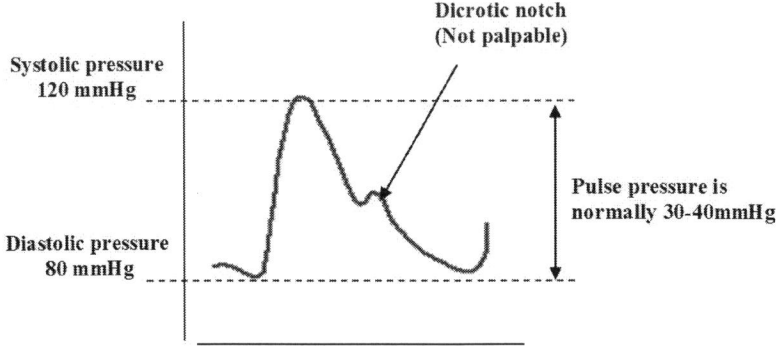

The arterial pulse is the activity of the left ventricle expressed in dilatation and subsequent contraction of the arterial wall

- The pulse normally reflects the **rate** and **rhythm** of contraction and relaxation of the heart.

- Pulse is commonly measured at the wrist where the artery passes over the radius or at the carotid artery in the neck just lateral to the thyroid cartilage (Best for assessing **character and volume**).

- **Volume** refers to the power of the pulse which is dependent on stroke volume and is affected by cardiac lesions and other states, especially hypotension

- **Character** refers to how slowly or quickly the pulse achieves its power and is more indicative of valvular lesions. For example, note the general difference in character in the diagrams below.

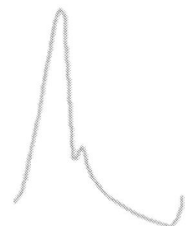

Bounding; high volume-
collapsing or waterhammer

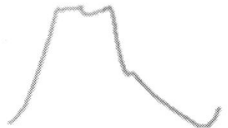

Plateau, weak or
low volume pulse

*Found in **aortic regurgitation**, severe anaemia etc. (see below). Note the increased pulse pressure.*

*Found in **aortic stenosis** due to the stiffness of the valve and consequent limitation of blood flow into the aorta.*

PALPATION OF PERIPHERAL PULSES AND ABNORMALITIES

Examination of arterial pulses enables assessment of heart rate, rhythm, volume and character of the pulse and assists in detection of blood flow obstruction.

Palpate with the pads of the index and middle fingers (or the thumb on larger pulses) and assess for 60 seconds.

Rate

- **Normal** - Pulse rate should be between **60 –80 bpm** in an adult sat quietly. Children may have higher pulse rates; athletes and elderly may be slower.

- **60-100** – Normal sinus rhythm (if abnormal, consider AV block or atrial flutter)

- **40-60** - Sinus bradycardia: Common in athletes. Hypothyroidism? Post MI? raised ICP?

- **<40** – Drug side effect (β-blockers)? heart block - consider idiopathic? Cardiomyopathy? Post MI complication?

- **>100** – Ventricular tachycardia? Sinus tachycardia - consider exercise? Anxiety? Anaemia? Thyrotoxicosis? Fever? Drugs (β_2 agonists e.g. salbutamol)? Heart failure? Hypovolaemic shock (e.g. GIT bleeding)?

Rhythm

- **Regularly irregular** – Inspiratory increase, i.e. sinus arrhythmia (Normal in young – subtler and less noticeable with age)? Digoxin toxicity? Heart block?

- **Irregularly irregular** – Atrial fibrillation (Test for *pulse deficit* i.e. palpate and auscultate together)? Multiple extra-systole? For both consider ischaemic heart disease. Drugs? Thyrotoxicosis?

Character and Volume (Realms of cardiology but may assess plateau, low volume, high volume/collapsing - see diagram above)

- *Normal* – Pulse smooth and rounded, pulse pressure 30–40 mmHg (NB Pulse pressure – widens with age due to arteriosclerosis i.e. reduced distensibility of arteries causes rise in systolic pressure).

- *Plateau pulse* (Slow rising, small volume) – Aortic stenosis.

- *Low volume* – Mitral stenosis? Hypovolaemia (shock)? Pulmonary hypertension?

- *High volume and collapsing* (aka. bounding, waterhammer)

  If detected, hold the patient's arm above their shoulder to test further, which will cause it to becomes more prominent. Occurs in:

  i) Increased stroke volume states, e.g. aortic regurgitation, severe anaemia, fever, thyrotoxicosis, AV defects, pregnancy.

ii) Increased stroke volume due to bradycardia and complete heart block.

iii) Decreased compliance of aortic walls as in ageing or atherosclerosis.

Get to know the next 4 when you are fully familiar with the above.

- **Bisferiens pulse** (Increased pulse with a double systolic peak) - Aortic regurgitation or combined aortic regurgitation and stenosis

- **Dicrotic pulse** (Carotid pulse with exaggerated dicrotic wave) – Typhoid fever.

- **Pulsus alternans** (Alternating high and low volume beats) – Left ventricular failure (Confirmed by sphygmomanometry; usually accompanied by S3)

- **Pulsus paradoxus** (Volume severely decreases on inspiration) – Cardiac tamponade? Constrictive pericarditis? Severe airways obstruction?

Inequality between radial pulses – Dissecting aortic aneurysm.

Radio-femoral delay – Coarctation of the aorta.

Sites of major pulse points and some disease indications

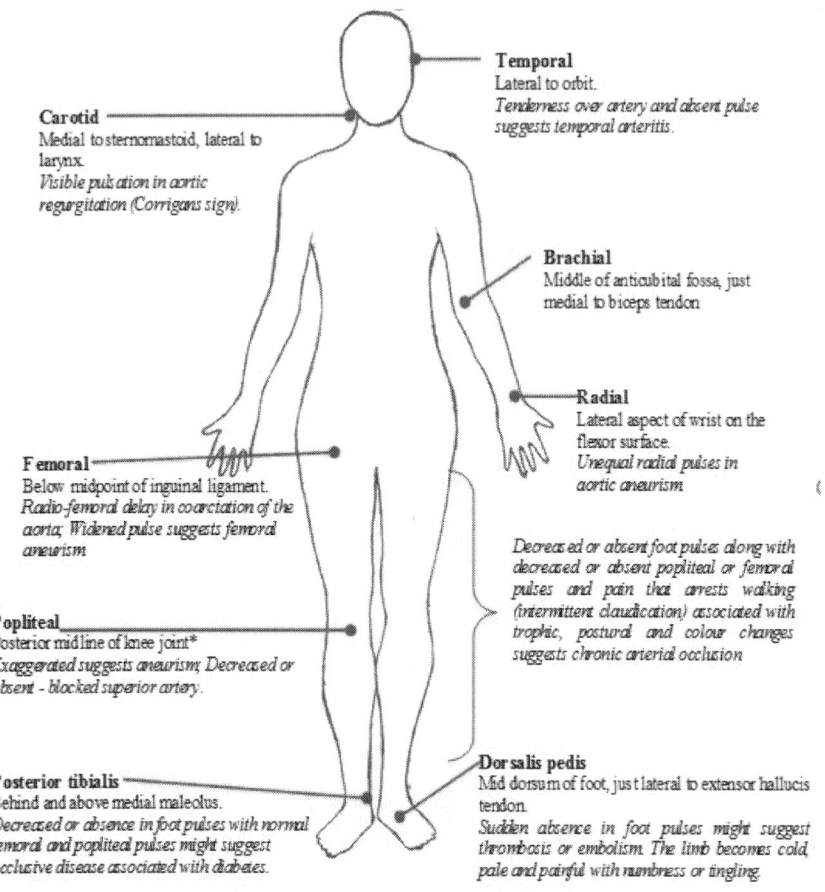

Temporal
Lateral to orbit.
Tenderness over artery and absent pulse suggests temporal arteritis.

Carotid
Medial to sternomastoid, lateral to larynx.
Visible pulsation in aortic regurgitation (Corrigans sign).

Brachial
Middle of anticubital fossa, just medial to biceps tendon

Radial
Lateral aspect of wrist on the flexor surface.
Unequal radial pulses in aortic aneurism

Femoral
Below midpoint of inguinal ligament.
Radio-femoral delay in coarctation of the aorta; Widened pulse suggests femoral aneurism

Decreased or absent foot pulses along with decreased or absent popliteal or femoral pulses and pain that arrests walking (intermittent claudication) associated with trophic, postural and colour changes suggests chronic arterial occlusion

Popliteal
Posterior midline of knee joint*
Exaggerated suggests aneurism; Decreased or absent - blocked superior artery.

Posterior tibialis
Behind and above medial maleolus.
Decreased or absence in foot pulses with normal femoral and popliteal pulses might suggest occlusive disease associated with diabetes.

Dorsalis pedis
Mid dorsum of foot, just lateral to extensor hallucis tendon.
Sudden absence in foot pulses might suggest thrombosis or embolism. The limb becomes cold, pale and painful with numbness or tingling.

* Press both fingers into a slightly flexed and relaxed joint (more deep and diffuse than other pulses).

APENDIX 2.   BLOOD PRESSURE

What is blood pressure?

- When the heart pumps blood it creates a pressure in the arteries called blood pressure (BP).

- The pressure is greatest when the heart muscle is contracting and lowest when it is relaxing.

- The contraction pressure is known as <u>systolic</u> and the relaxation pressure is known as <u>diastolic</u>.

- Systolic pressure reflects how hard the left ventricle is working to pump blood around the body. Several factors can increase the contraction effort of the heart, e.g. Stress / anxiety, exercise, increased resistance of blood vessels, blood viscosity, increased volume of blood, etc.

- Diastolic pressure reflects the resistance of the small arteries and capillaries to blood flow and therefore, the load against which the heart must work. If resistance is high, so is diastolic pressure.

SIMPLIFIED DIAGRAM OF FACTORS AFFECTING BP

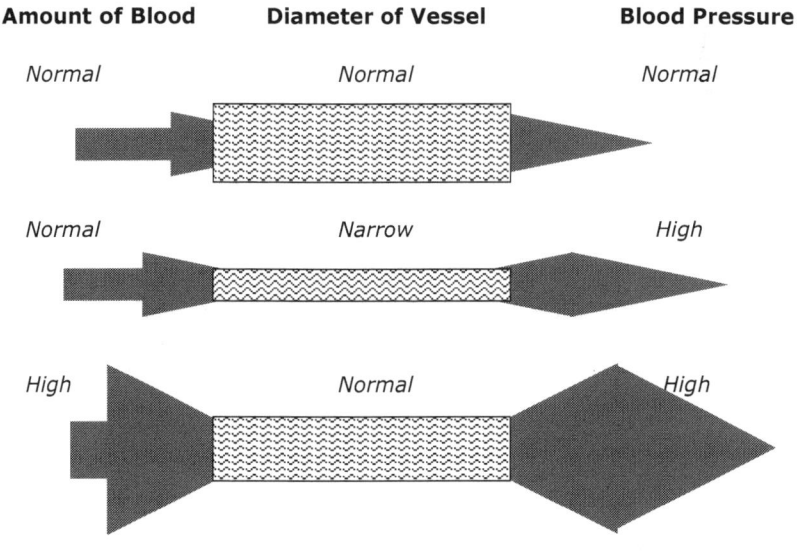

Amount of Blood	Diameter of Vessel	Blood Pressure
Normal	Normal	Normal
Normal	Narrow	High
High	Normal	High

Measurement of blood pressure

- Until relatively recently, BP was measured using a mercury (**Hg**) filled pressure gauge or sphygmomanometer (**manometer** – instrument for measuring fluid pressures) in millimetre (**mm**) graduations: hence, it was measured in **mmHg**.

- The applied cuff of the monitor is inflated 30mmHg above the **palpable** estimated systolic pressure to ensure complete occlusion of the artery and to prevent incorrect estimation, particularly due to **auscultatory gap**.

- The cuff is then slowly deflated and the brachial artery auscultated for the Korotkoff sounds that indicate systolic and diastolic pressure.

Note
So-called "white-coat hypertension" (occurs due to clinical situations) is a confounding issue in sphygmomanometry and in the past (and perhaps even now) was a cause of an inappropriate diagnosis of hypertension.

This is no less of an issue in the relaxed atmosphere of the herbal clinic and you should always consider this issue when you are estimating blood pressure.

Notes on Hypertension (Abnormally high arterial BP)

Some useful basic points to consider:

- Systolic pressure is governed by i) cardiac activity ii) elasticity and distensibility of arteries. Therefore:

BP = Cardiac Output X Total Peripheral Resistance

- Ageing is associated with arteriosclerosis (hardening of the arteries). This results in increased systolic and diastolic pressure, i.e. it is like forcing blood through a solid pipe rather than through a hose that will expand and contract with changing pressure.

- High Blood Pressure increases the risk of cardiovascular disease e.g.

    1. **Left Ventricular Hypertrophy** - resulting in Heart Failure

    2. **Ischaemic Heart Disease -** resulting in Heart Failure

    3. **Stroke** - Cerebral haemorrhage or infarction.

- You should always consider how case history is affecting the physiological mechanism controlling BP

Physiological mechanisms controlling BP

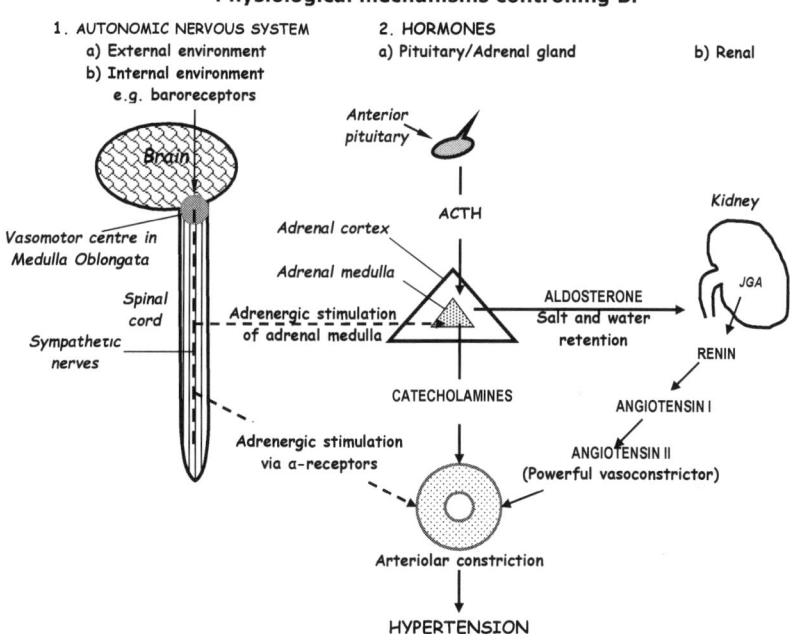

Diagram adapted from Macfarlane et al (2000)

1. a) *External factors such as stress and anxiety can result in increased sympathetic production of adrenalin b) baroreceptors are responsible for minute-to-minute regulation of BP but baroreflex may fail or be reset in certain circumstances. 2. a) Increased production of ACTH (e.g. due stress) results in increased aldosterone production with consequent sodium/water retention and b) activation of the renin-angiotensin system.*

Types of Hypertension

- **Essential (aka. Primary) hypertension** – 90-95% of cases have no obvious cause. Possibly due to vascular changes resulting from sympathetic over activity, thus resetting baroreceptors.

- **Secondary Hypertension** – 5-10% of cases are a complication of other diseases, e.g.

  - Kidney disease - chronic renal failure, renal artery stenosis, diabetic nephropathy, polycystic kidneys. (The mechanism is usually renal ischaemia).

  - Endocrine disorders – Cushing's syndrome (corticosteroid excess); Conn's syndrome (aldosterone excess); phaeochromocytoma (adrenaline excess).

  - Coarctation of the aorta.

  - Pregnancy – eclampsia.

  - Drugs – steroids, contraceptive pill.

BP Classification

Be aware that classifications vary but a rough guide to estimating normal systolic BP might be:

1. 15-25 years of the age: 100 + age.

2. Over 25 years of age: 110 plus half the age

BP Classification		
	SYSTOLIC	**DIASTOLIC**
Optimal	<120	<80
Normal	<130	<88
High normal	130-139	85-89
Mild hypertension	140-145	90-99
Moderate hypertension	160-179	100-109
Severe hypertension	≥180	≥ 100
Malignant hypertension	210	120

When you have estimated the patient's BP, keep in mind that:

- Systolic pressure reflects LV contraction.

- Diastolic pressure provides information about vascular resistance.

- Pulse pressure (Systolic – Diastolic) provides information about the cardiovascular system, e.g. conditions such as atherosclerosis and PDA, which greatly increase pulse pressure (An average pulse pressure is around 40mmHg).

Notes on Hypotension

- Hypotension can be broadly defined as blood pressure below the normal expected for an individual in a given environment.

- People with 'normal' low blood pressure, on average, tend to live longer. In a small minority (i.e. cases below < 90/60 mmHg) with an underlying cause, treatment may be necessary due to inadequate blood flow to vital organs such as the heart and brain.

- Hypotension is an indicator of lowered contractility, hypovolaemia, abnormal vasodilatation, or occlusion/blockage

- Common pathologies resulting in hypotension are:

  o Myocardial ischaemia/infarction.

  o Sepsis (overwhelming infection, usually by bacteria).

  o Hypovolaemia secondary to bleeding.

- Other causes of low blood pressure:

  o BP lowering drugs – e.g. alpha blockers, such as doxazosin may cause a drop upon standing.

- Rare diseases of the nerves that control the reflexes in the veins, i.e. veins do not contract (as normal) on standing resulting in severe BP reduction.

- Increasing age – hardening arteries may occasionally cause a fall in blood pressure when standing.

- Adrenal failure – results in excess sodium excretion and consequent water loss resulting in hypovolaemia.

CONCLUDING REMARKS

These notes are for use by practitioners trained or training under the guidance of an organised programme of study such as that qualified by the National Institute of Medical Herbalists or similar body. They can serve as a quick reference to orthodox clinical examination skills to support one's chosen 'traditional' methods. In addition, knowledge of these skills will ensure safe diagnosis and prevent possibly flawed over-reliance on traditional methods when orthodox diagnosis and treatment might be necessary.

However, to prevent over-reliance on this essential knowledge alone, and by doing so diminishing the sanity of our Herbalist/Naturopathic paradigms (or at worst, totally succumbing to the 'dark side' ☺), it is worth remembering Hamlet's admonition to his friend that "*There are more things in heaven and earth, Horatio, than are dreamt of in our philosophy.*"

But perhaps a final word from my friend Elwood P. Dowd.

"*Well, I've wrestled with reality for 35 years, Doctor, and I'm happy to state I finally won over it*"

ABOUT THE AUTHOR

Peter is a Medical Herbalist (retired) who trained under the auspices of The National Institute of Medical Herbalists, of which he is a member. Prior to retirement, he operated successful practices in Lytham St Annes and Poulton le Fylde, Lancashire and lectured in Physiology, Medical Science and other Biosciences at Blackpool and the Fylde College. For several years, he taught Clinical Skills to undergraduate Medical Herbalists at The University of Central Lancashire. He holds honours degrees in Herbal Medicine and Health Science for which his final thesis was 'Qigong: A Scientific Perspective' since published in the *Qi Journal.*

He believes that medicine is like a precious gem that should not be squandered and so is a strong advocate for avoiding unnecessary medical intervention. He encourages personal responsibility for health and promotes practices that engender physical and mental wellbeing and reduce overreliance on external medical intervention. An essential element of his treatments incorporated complete nutrition and bodywork / relaxation-meditation methods, including aspects of Chinese Internal Arts, which he has studied and practiced for more than 40 years. He is one of the founding members of the Fylde Tai Chi Association, a local organisation that promotes the regular practice of Tai Chi and related methods. With his brother, John, he is co-author of 'Understanding Chi Kung'.

BIBLIOGRAPHY

Bickley, L.S. (1999), <u>Bates Guide to Clinical Examination and History Taking</u>. Philadelphia: Lippincott Williams & Wilkins.

Cox & Roper (2005) <u>Clinical Skills</u>. Oxford University Press.

Kumar & Clark (1994), <u>Clinical Medicine</u>. London: W.B. Saunders.

Macfarlane, Reid & Callander (2000) <u>Pathology Illustrated</u>. Harcourt Publishers (Churchill Livingstone): London.

Printed in Great Britain
by Amazon